THE NEW DIVERTICULITIS DIET COOKBOOK FOR BEGINNERS

A Simple Nutritional Guide for Symptom Relief, Reducing Inflammation, Improving Digestion, and Alleviating Pain and Flare-Ups

Michael Slowick, RDN

COPYRIGHT PAGE

Copyright © 2024 Michael Slowick, RDN. All rights reserved.

No part of this publication or work may be copied, stored in a retrieval system, or transmitted in any form or by any means without prior written permission from the publisher or author, or through payment of the appropriate per-copy fee to the copyright holder, except as permitted under Sections 107 or 108 of the United States Copyright Act of 1976, or as expressly allowed by law, license, or terms agreed upon with the relevant reprographics rights organization.

The publisher and author expressly disclaim any implied guarantees of merchantability and fitness for a particular purpose. While every effort has been made to ensure the accuracy of the information provided herein, no promises are made regarding its completeness or accuracy. Any statements made by sales employees or representatives, whether verbal or written, do not constitute extended or implied guarantees.

Table of Contents

COPYRIGHT PAGE 2

Table of Contents 4

CHAPTER I: INTRODUCTION TO DIVERTICULITIS 1

Let's Get Real About Diverticulitis: Understanding Diverticulitis 3

Recognizing the Telltale Signs: Causes and Risk Factors 7

Looking Out for Tell-Tale Signs: Symptoms and Diagnosis 10

Getting the Lowdown on Treatment Options: Treating Diverticulitis 17

CHAPTER II: STAGES OF DIVERTICULITIS 23

Recommended Diet during Diverticulitis 26

Transitioning in Each Phase 30

Weighty Matters: Managing Weight with Diverticulitis 34

Alcohol and Diverticulitis: Navigating Alcohol with Care 37

Supplements, Herbs and Alternate Treatments for Diverticulitis Support: Separating Fact from Fiction 40

CHAPTER III: A DEEP DIVE INTO DIVERTICULITIS NUTRITION 50

Food as Medicine: Importance of Diet in Managing Diverticulitis 52

The Nutritional Puzzle: Goals of a Diverticulitis Diet 56

Why Your Diet Matters More Than You Think: Benefits of a Well-Planned Diet 59

CHAPTER IV: MAKING SENSE OF FOOD CHOICES 64

High-Fiber Foods: Your Gut's Greatest Allies 71

Low-Fiber Fare: Foods to Limit or Avoid 84

Extra One Week Meal Plan 88

Grocery Guides: Stocking Your Pantry with Success 94

Meal Planning Resources: Practical Tools for Meal Planning 99

CHAPTER V: HEALTHY DIVERTICULITIS-FRIENDLY RECIPES 101

DIVERTICULITIS-FRIENDLY CLEAR LIQUID DIET 101

Lemon Ginger Herbal Tea 101

Chicken Broth Soup 102

Apple Juice Jelly 103

Clear Veggie Broth 104

Refreshing Grape Juice Slushie 105

Herbal Peppermint Tea 105

Clear Vegetable Soup 106

Pineapple Juice Jelly 107

Green Tea with Honey 108

Watermelon Juice Slushie 109

Clear Chicken Broth 109

Clear Vegetable Broth 110

DIVERTICULITIS-FRIENDLY HIGH FIBER SOUPS 112

Slow Cooker Lentil, Sausage and Kale Soup 112

Smooth Broccoli Soup 114

Pea and Pesto Soup 116

Creamy Carrot Soup 117

Creamy Carrot Soup 119

Mushroom and Ginger Soup 121

Kidney Bean Soup 122

Creamy Squash Soup.. 124

Creamy Chickpea Soup... 126

Cannellini and Butter Bean Soup............................ 127

Beef and Vegetable Soup.. 128

Beans with Greens Soup 130

Vegetable and Lentil Stew 132

DIVERTICULITIS-FRIENDLY SALAD RECIPES ... 134

Asian Chicken Salad 134

Tuna Cakes and Smashed Potatoes....................... 135

Bean and Couscous Salad 137

Brown Rice Greek Salad... 138

Cilantro Bean Salad.. 140

Fruit Salad with Avocado 141

Garbanzo and Tomato Salad 143

Greek White Bean and Feta Salad 144

Green Bean Potato Salad 146

Green Bean Tuna Salad 147

Grilled Shrimp and Bean Salad 149

Light Shrimp and Barley Salad 151

Mango Black Bean Salad 152

Mediterranean Salmon and Potato Salad 153

Quick Spinach and Black Bean Salad 155

Shrimp, Pasta and Spinach Salad 156

DIVERTICULITIS-FRIENDLY HIGH FIBER RECIPES 158

Apple Chicken Pita Pocket 158

Baked Salmon with Vegetable Quinoa 159

Grilled Chicken Breast with Mashed Potatoes and Steamed Carrot 161

Apple and Pear Pita Pockets 163

Apple Raisin Pancakes 164

Apricot Honey Oatmeal 166

Asparagus and Bean Frittata 167

Banana Bran Muffins 169

Banana Breakfast Smoothie 170

Bran Muffins 171

Breakfast Carrot Cake 174

Broccoli Omelet 176

Carrot and Zucchini Bread 177

Pumpkin Pie Oatmeal 179

Santé Fe Omelet 180

Sunrise Burrito Wrap 182

Tropical Fruit Smoothie 184

Zucchini and Bean Scramble 185

DIVERTICULITIS-FRIENDLY HEALTHY SNACKS 187

Baked Sweet Potato Fries 187

Citrus Carrots 188

Greek Lettuce Wraps 189

Honey Baked Apples 190

Kidney Bean Salsa 192

Oatmeal Chocolate Chip Cookies 193

White Bean Puree 194

Baked Artichoke Dip 195

Spinach and Mushroom Toss 197

CHAPTER VI: BEYOND THE PLATE: LIFESTYLE STRATEGIES FOR DIVERTICULITIS MANAGEMENT 199

Move It or Lose It: Exercise Essentials 204

Stress Less, Live More: Stress Management Techniques 207

CHAPTER VII: BEFORE YOU GO, HERE'S A FINAL REMINDER! 213

Finding Support and Community along the Way:
Seeking Guidance.. 220

CHAPTER I: INTRODUCTION TO DIVERTICULITIS

Diverticulitis occurs when the small pockets inside your colon, known as diverticula, become inflamed. This condition, called diverticulosis, is quite common, especially with age, and most people never experience any issues with it. However, if one of these diverticula becomes inflamed, it can lead to acute pain and other symptoms, potentially indicating an infection that requires medical attention.

Although diverticulosis is prevalent, diverticulitis is a less common complication, affecting around 4% of individuals with diverticulosis. Once you've had an episode, there's a 20% chance of recurrence. While rare in the past, diverticular disease has become increasingly common in Western societies, encompassing various digestive tract conditions.

Among these conditions, diverticulitis is the most serious, potentially causing discomfort and, in severe cases, complications. **If left untreated, these complications can result in long-term health issues.** Healthcare professionals *classify diverticulitis based on whether it's acute or chronic and whether it's complicated or uncomplicated.*

Acute diverticulitis typically arises suddenly and resolves shortly with treatment, though some individuals experience recurring episodes or develop chronic inflammation. The reasons for this can vary, from incomplete healing of an acute episode to underlying chronic colon conditions.

In most cases, diverticulitis is uncomplicated, involving inflammation and potential infection that can be easily treated. However, it becomes complicated when inflammation leads to secondary issues. For instance, severe acute inflammation might cause a diverticulum to rupture, while chronic inflammation could result in scarring.

Let's Get Real About Diverticulitis: Understanding Diverticulitis

The large bowel or large intestine, commonly known as the colon, is a vital organ in the human digestive system. This system comprises organs that enable us to consume food and utilize it to energize our bodies.

The colon plays a crucial role in processing the food we eat. Here's how food progresses through our system:

Food begins its journey in the mouth, where it's broken down by teeth into smaller pieces. Once swallowed, it travels through the esophagus and into the stomach.

In the stomach, food undergoes further breakdown into liquid form before moving into the small bowel or intestine.

Within the small bowel, aided by the pancreas, liver, and gallbladder, food breakdown continues, and essential vitamins and nutrients are absorbed.

Remaining liquid material proceeds into the colon, where water absorption occurs. Bacteria in the colon further break down the remaining material. The colon then transports this leftover material into the rectum.

The rectum acts as a storage reservoir for waste. Muscles in the rectum facilitate the expulsion of waste, termed stool, from the body through the anus.

Maintaining a healthy diet is crucial for overall well-being, particularly for a healthy colon. **A diet low in calories yet high in fiber, primarily consisting of fruits and vegetables, is essential.** Additionally, regular exercise and healthy lifestyle choices, such as moderating alcohol intake and avoiding smoking, contribute significantly to good colon health. **When the colon functions improperly, it can lead to issues like bloating, gas, pain, constipation, or diarrhea.**

Diverticulosis manifests when small pouches, known as diverticula, form and protrude through weakened areas in the colon wall, primarily in the sigmoid colon, the lower part of the colon.

A single pouch is termed a diverticulum, while multiple pouches are referred to as diverticula. Many individuals with diverticula experience no symptoms or complications. However, in some instances, these pouches may cause symptoms or inflammation.

Diverticulitis arises when diverticula become inflamed, sometimes suddenly, and can lead to severe complications.

Diverticular disease encompasses various conditions including chronic symptoms, diverticular bleeding, and complications of diverticulitis.

Recognizing the Telltale Signs: Causes and Risk Factors

Diverticula can form when weakened areas in your colon give in, leading to small pouches protruding through the colon wall. Diverticulitis occurs when these pouches tear, causing inflammation and sometimes infection.

The exact reason why some individuals develop diverticulitis while others do not remains unclear to doctors. However, research indicates that genetics may play a role. Interestingly, many people with diverticulitis are unaware of their condition.

The likelihood of experiencing diverticulitis increases with age, particularly after 40. Several risk factors contribute to its development:

- Being overweight
- Smoking
- Lack of physical activity
- Consuming a diet high in fat and red meat but low in fiber
- Taking certain medications, including steroids, opioids, and nonsteroidal anti-inflammatory drugs like ibuprofen or naproxen

The exact causes of diverticulosis and diverticular disease remain unclear. However, epidemiological studies have identified certain factors linked to a higher risk of developing these conditions. Often, discussions about these risk factors lack precision in distinguishing between different aspects.

It's important to recognize that risk factors for diverticulosis, diverticulitis, diverticular perforation, and bleeding from diverticula should be considered separately. For instance, dietary fiber has been extensively studied as both a risk and protective factor for diverticulosis and related ailments. Recent research has challenged the long-standing belief that a high-fiber diet guards against diverticula formation, yet it's crucial not to overlook the strong evidence supporting its protective role against diverticular disease.

While **some risk factors like age, gender, and genetics are beyond our control, lifestyle choices regarding diet, alcohol intake, and physical activity can be influential.** Additionally, comorbidities and medications play significant roles in the development of diverticulitis, perforation, or bleeding. Thoroughly assessing a patient's medical history can help mitigate risks by opting for less harmful medications and guiding treatment decisions based on specific health conditions.

Looking Out for Tell-Tale Signs: Symptoms and Diagnosis

Symptoms

Symptoms of diverticulitis *typically include intense abdominal pain and fever.* The pain can range from sharp and piercing to a burning sensation and is often moderate to severe. This discomfort may persist for days, primarily concentrated on the lower left side of the abdomen, although in individuals of Asian descent, it might occasionally be more pronounced on the right side.

Diverticulitis can manifest in acute or chronic forms. Acute episodes involve severe attacks of infection and inflammation, while chronic cases may see a reduction in inflammation and infection but never complete resolution. Prolonged inflammation can lead to bowel obstruction, resulting in symptoms like constipation, thin stools, diarrhea, bloating, and abdominal pain. If the obstruction persists, abdominal pain and tenderness may worsen, accompanied by nausea and vomiting.

Common indicators of diverticulitis include constant, prolonged abdominal pain, usually on the lower left side, though sometimes on the right side, especially in those of Asian descent. Other signs include nausea, vomiting, fever, abdominal tenderness, and bowel irregularities like constipation or diarrhea.

Diagnosing

The symptoms of diverticulitis can resemble those of other conditions, so your doctor will aim to narrow down the possibilities by excluding other potential issues. This typically begins with *a physical examination*, which may also involve a pelvic exam for women. Following this initial assessment, your doctor may request one or more tests, which can include:

To diagnose diverticular disease, doctors typically review your medical history, conduct a physical examination, and order relevant tests. In some instances, doctors may observe pouches in the colon wall during tests such as x-rays or colonoscopies conducted for other reasons. If these pouches are present without accompanying symptoms, your doctor may diagnose diverticulosis rather than diverticular disease.

When gathering your medical history, your doctor will inquire about your symptoms, bowel habits, dietary intake, existing medical conditions, and current medications.

During the physical exam, your doctor may:

- Check your blood pressure, heart rate, and temperature.
- Palpate your abdomen to detect tenderness or masses.
- Listen to abdominal sounds using a stethoscope.
- Additionally, a digital rectal exam may also be performed as part of the assessment.

Doctors employ various tests to diagnose diverticular disease, which may include blood tests, stool tests, imaging studies, and colonoscopies. These diagnostic tools help provide a comprehensive understanding of your condition and guide appropriate treatment decisions.

1. **Blood Tests:**

A healthcare professional will draw a blood sample from you and send it to a laboratory for analysis. Blood tests are commonly used by doctors to detect signs of diverticulitis or its associated complications.

2. **Stool Test:**

Doctors may request a stool test to determine whether you have diverticular disease or another gastrointestinal issue like irritable bowel syndrome. Your doctor will provide you with a container to collect a stool sample and give instructions on where to send or take the sample for testing.

3. **Imaging Tests:**

Doctors often diagnose diverticular disease using imaging tests such as:

i. *Computed Tomography (CT):* This method combines x-rays and computer technology to generate detailed images of your internal organs.

ii. *Ultrasound*: Utilizing sound waves, ultrasound creates images of your organs.

iii. *Magnetic Resonance Imaging (MRI)*: MRI captures images of your body's internal organs and soft tissues without the use of x-rays.

4. **Colonoscopy**:

A colonoscopy may be recommended by doctors to confirm a diverticular disease diagnosis and exclude other conditions like cancer. Additionally, doctors may order a colonoscopy to identify and manage diverticular bleeding.

During a colonoscopy, doctors utilize a colonoscope, a long, flexible tube equipped with a light and a small camera on one end, to examine the rectum and colon lining.

Getting the Lowdown on Treatment Options: Treating Diverticulitis

If diverticulitis is mild and uncomplicated, *it may resolve on its own*, but it's crucial to seek evaluation from a healthcare provider. They may prescribe antibiotics to address any infection and provide prescription pain relief if necessary. Additionally, your provider will offer guidance on home care during your recovery, which typically takes about a week. It's important to stay in touch with your provider during this time.

If your healthcare provider approves, you can manage diverticulitis at home by:

Following a liquid diet: Avoiding solid foods allows your bowels to rest and recuperate. Your provider can offer specific dietary recommendations.

Taking prescription antibiotics if required: The type of antibiotic prescribed will depend on the nature of the infection.

Using acetaminophen for pain relief: Over-the-counter pain relievers like acetaminophen are preferred, as other options may increase the risk of gastrointestinal bleeding.

If you experience **RECTAL BLEEDING**, even in small amounts, it's important to seek medical attention promptly. While some cases of diverticular bleeding may resolve spontaneously, others may require intervention. Doctors may employ procedures such as:

Colonoscopy: This procedure allows a doctor to use specialized tools inserted through a colonoscope to halt bleeding.

Angiogram: An angiogram, a type of x-ray using dye to visualize blood vessels, can help locate bleeding vessels in the colon. During this procedure, a radiologist may inject medications or other substances to stop bleeding.

Surgery: In some cases, surgical intervention may be necessary to address diverticular bleeding.

Doctors typically manage the complications of diverticular disease in a hospital setting. For **ABSCESSES**, different treatment approaches may be recommended:

- Antibiotics are often prescribed for small abscesses.
- Larger abscesses or those unresponsive to antibiotics may require drainage.
- Surgery might be advised after the resolution of a large abscess to prevent recurrence.

For other complications of diverticulitis, such as **FISTULAS, INTESTINAL OBSTRUCTION,**

PERFORATION, OR PERITONITIS, surgery is commonly recommended.

In certain cases, doctors may suggest lifestyle modifications or surgical interventions to prevent diverticulitis. Research indicates that specific lifestyle habits may reduce the risk of developing diverticulitis, including:

- Consuming a high-fiber, low-red meat diet
- Engaging in regular physical activity
- Quitting smoking, if applicable
- Achieving and maintaining a healthy weight

Discuss with your doctor whether implementing these lifestyle changes could help lower your risk of diverticulitis. If you've had diverticulitis in the past, consult with your doctor about the potential benefits of lifestyle adjustments in reducing the risk of recurrence. Additionally, discuss your medication regimen with your doctor to ascertain if any medications might increase your risk of diverticulitis.

Surgery may be considered in certain cases, especially after a person has experienced uncomplicated diverticulitis. This surgical intervention involves removing a portion of the colon to prevent future occurrences of diverticulitis. The decision to proceed with surgery depends on various factors, including the individual's diverticulitis history, overall health, and other relevant considerations.

CHAPTER II: STAGES OF DIVERTICULITIS

Hinchey and his team introduced a comprehensive categorization system for diverticulitis, delineating it into four distinct stages:

In **Stage I**, the condition is *marked by the formation of a pericolic abscess*, a localized collection of pus, typically confined within the mesentery of the colon. This stage represents an initial inflammatory response, often characterized by localized pain and tenderness in the abdominal region.

Advancing to **Stage II**, the scenario becomes more intricate with the *emergence of a pelvic abscess*. This occurs as a consequence of the perforation of a pericolic abscess, leading to the accumulation of infectious material within the pelvic cavity. Here, the abscess may find itself encapsulated by neighboring anatomical structures such as the colon, mesocolon, omentum, small bowel, and even reproductive organs like the uterus, fallopian tubes, and ovaries, alongside the pelvic peritoneum. This stage often presents with more pronounced symptoms, including severe abdominal pain and potential signs of infection such as fever and elevated white blood cell count.

Stage III denotes a critical juncture, where the condition *escalates to generalized peritonitis*. This occurs when either a pericolic or pelvic abscess ruptures, spilling its contents into the free peritoneal cavity. The peritoneum, the protective lining of the abdominal cavity, becomes inflamed and infected, resulting in widespread abdominal tenderness, rigidity, and often systemic signs of sepsis.

Stage IV represents the *most severe manifestation, characterized by fecal peritonitis.* Here, a diverticulum—small pouches that form in the weakened areas of the colon—undergoes uncontrolled perforation, releasing fecal matter directly into the peritoneal cavity. This stage is associated with a profound systemic inflammatory response, marked by severe abdominal pain, septic shock, and a high risk of life-threatening complications such as multiple organ failure.

The Hinchey classification system provides a comprehensive framework for understanding the progression and severity of diverticulitis, guiding clinicians in determining appropriate management strategies tailored to the specific stage of the disease.

Recommended Diet during Diverticulitis

Clear Liquid Diet:

When diagnosed with diverticulitis, healthcare providers often recommend a brief stint on *a clear liquid diet lasting 1 to 2 days*. This regimen serves to **give the gastrointestinal tract a chance to recuperate and mend.**

Clear liquids encompass a range of options such as water, sports drinks, transparent broth, tea, flavored gelatin, clear juice-based frozen ice pops, black coffee, and fruit juices without pulp like cranberry, grape, and apple.

During this phase, it's advisable to consume 1 to 2 items from this list every few hours, rather than adhering to a conventional meal schedule. However, it's essential to note that this dietary restriction is temporary. After a day or two of clear liquids, individuals typically progress to reintroducing solid foods.

Low-Fiber Diet:

Following a brief period on a clear liquid diet, transitioning to a low-fiber diet is often the next step, particularly in cases of uncomplicated diverticulitis where inflammation exists without abscesses or tears in the intestinal wall.

This regimen *involves limiting intake of whole grains and opting for alternatives like white bread, white-flour tortillas, crackers, refined cereal, pasta, or white rice.* Additionally, the low-fiber diet incorporates easily digestible options such as applesauce, canned fruit, or soft, peeled fruits, thoroughly cooked vegetables, lean poultry, fish, eggs, and smooth nut butters. Dairy products like cheese, milk, and yogurt are also permissible.

High-Fiber Diet:

Once the *episode of diverticulitis has subsided, individuals can gradually return to a regular diet.* However, the focus shifts to adopting a dietary pattern conducive to long-term well-being.

According to recommendations from the **American Gastroenterological Association (AGA), a fiber-rich diet is encouraged for individuals with diverticulosis**, and this holds true even for those with a history of diverticulitis.

While concrete evidence on the role of fiber in preventing diverticulitis is somewhat lacking, AGA guidelines emphasize the overall health benefits associated with a high-fiber diet. Moreover, there is no explicit recommendation to avoid nuts and popcorn, as studies have not established a definitive link between these foods and an increased risk of diverticulitis.

A Word of Caution

Diverticulitis warrants prompt medical attention, often involving antibiotic therapy and, in severe cases, surgical intervention. Dietary adjustments play a crucial role in managing the condition, but it's imperative to seek guidance from healthcare professionals regarding the most suitable short and long-term dietary strategies. Given the potential for diverticulitis to precipitate severe complications, individuals should promptly seek medical care if they experience persistent or severe abdominal pain, fever, chills, or rectal bleeding. Additionally, any notable changes in bowel habits, persistent vomiting, bloating, or nausea should be promptly reported to a healthcare provider for further evaluation and management.

Transitioning in Each Phase

During a bout of diverticulitis, it's often necessary to allow your bowel some time to recuperate. This typically entails consuming only clear liquids for a few days.

Liquid Diet:

The initial phase of managing a diverticulitis flare-up involves specific foods, such as broth, fruit juices without pulp like apple juice, gelatin, ice chips, ice pops devoid of fruit bits or pulp, tea or coffee sans cream, and water. However, a liquid diet should only be adhered to for a brief period before progressing to the next phase.

Recovery Diet:

Upon transitioning from the liquid diet, a low-fiber or low-residue diet, also termed a soft diet, is recommended during the recovery phase. This temporary healing diet comprises various food categories:

- Starchy foods like white bread, white rice, and potatoes without skin.
- Dairy products such as milk and cottage cheese.

- Protein sources like eggs, fish, lean poultry, yogurt, and gelatin.
- Fruit options including applesauce, canned or cooked fruit, and fruit juice without pulp.
- Well-cooked vegetables.
- Broth and ice pops.

Foods to Avoid:

During the recovery period, it's advisable to steer clear of high-fiber foods like beans and legumes, whole grains and whole-grain products, nuts and seeds, raw or dried fruits or juices with pulp, uncooked vegetables, potato skins, processed meats, crunchy peanut butter, and fried or spicy foods.

Gradual Increase in Fiber:

After recuperating from a diverticulitis episode, healthcare providers typically recommend gradually reintroducing fiber into your diet. Increasing fiber intake, either through dietary sources or supplements, can aid in preventing future flare-ups. Fiber softens stool and alleviates constipation, thereby reducing pressure in the colon and potentially preventing future diverticulitis episodes.

Fluid Intake:

As you incorporate more fiber into your diet, it's essential to pay attention to your fluid intake. Fiber requires adequate hydration to function effectively. Insufficient water consumption can result in overly firm stools, making them difficult to pass.

Meal Timing:

Some individuals with digestive issues, including diverticular disease, find relief by consuming smaller, more frequent meals rather than three larger meals per day. However, there's no universal recommendation for meal timing with diverticular disease. Finding the optimal meal timing and portion sizes may require experimentation to determine what works best for you.

Weighty Matters: Managing Weight with Diverticulitis

In both acute and chronic instances of diverticulitis, it's common to experience a decrease in appetite, often accompanied by symptoms like fatigue and diminished performance. These indicators can sometimes serve as the initial warning signs that something may be amiss within your body.

Digestive ailments such as diverticulitis can induce sensations of nausea or abdominal discomfort, significantly dampening the desire to eat. Additionally, conditions like gastrointestinal infections, ulcers, gastritis (inflammation of the stomach lining), and pancreatitis (inflammation of the pancreas) can elicit similar symptoms of nausea or pain.

In severe cases of diverticulitis, the body may struggle to absorb an adequate amount of nutrients through the intestines, leading to undesirable weight loss.

If you find yourself experiencing a prolonged loss of appetite without an apparent cause and are shedding pounds unintentionally, it's crucial to seek medical attention promptly. It's especially imperative to consult a doctor if your weight loss is accompanied by other concerning symptoms such as:

- Abdominal pain or persistent headaches
- Indigestion or gastrointestinal discomfort
- Excessive thirst or unexplained fluctuations in fluid intake
- Fever and nocturnal perspiration
- Persistent feelings of exhaustion and lethargy
- Shortness of breath or difficulty breathing
- Persistent coughing or respiratory issues

Considering that obesity is a well-established risk factor for diverticulitis, weight management strategies, including weight loss when appropriate, are often recommended to mitigate the risk and manage the condition effectively.

Alcohol and Diverticulitis: Navigating Alcohol with Care

Several studies have explored the potential link between alcohol consumption and diverticular disease, yet the findings have been inconsistent.

While certain research indicates a notable association between alcohol consumption and diverticulosis, the exact mechanisms remain unclear. *Some theories propose that alcohol may induce dehydration, which in turn can lead* to hardened stools and heightened straining during bowel movements, thereby elevating the risk of diverticular formation.

Moreover, alcohol has been suggested to impede intestinal motility, potentially resulting in constipation and increased pressure within the intestines. This heightened pressure may exacerbate symptoms of diverticulitis and potentially contribute to more frequent flare-ups.

Given these considerations, individuals experiencing symptoms of diverticulitis are advised to consult their healthcare provider. Depending on individual circumstances, healthcare professionals may recommend abstaining from alcohol entirely to mitigate the progression of the condition. **It's generally prudent to refrain from alcohol consumption during**

diverticulitis episodes to minimize exacerbating symptoms.

Ethyl alcohol serves as the primary intoxicating component in alcoholic beverages, including beer, wine, and hard liquor. Should one choose to consume alcohol, it's essential to be mindful of the beverage's alcohol content.

Alcohol by volume (ABV) serves as a crucial metric for gauging a beverage's alcoholic potency, indicating the percentage of pure alcohol within its total volume.

For individuals grappling with alcohol abuse, abstaining from alcohol consumption can pose a significant challenge. Alcoholism, characterized by compulsive and excessive alcohol consumption despite adverse consequences, necessitates comprehensive treatment approaches such as alcohol rehabilitation programs. It's important to recognize that alcohol recovery constitutes a lifelong journey, with the potential for relapses. Resuming alcohol consumption, particularly after a period of abstinence, may precipitate or exacerbate diverticulitis symptoms, underscoring the importance of abstaining from alcohol in managing the condition.

Supplements, Herbs and Alternate Treatments for Diverticulitis Support: Separating Fact from Fiction

Food serves as the primary and most natural source of dietary fiber, yet individuals may opt for fiber supplements to boost their fiber intake. These supplements often contain insoluble fiber variants like psyllium and glucomannan, typically **recommended at doses ranging from 3 to 5 grams per day**. Additionally, **soluble fiber supplements such as flaxseed and oat bran, which are generally gentler on the digestive system**, may be advised by your healthcare provider. Consulting with your doctor can help determine the most suitable combination of supplements for your needs.

Glutamine, an amino acid naturally present in the body, plays a crucial role in maintaining intestinal health. Although evidence supporting its efficacy in alleviating diverticular disease symptoms is lacking, glutamine supplementation may contribute to overall gastrointestinal well-being. However, individuals with diabetes, seizures, liver conditions, or a history of manic episodes should avoid glutamine supplementation.

Omega-3 fatty acids, abundant in fish oil, exhibit anti-inflammatory properties and may aid in combating inflammation associated with diverticulitis. Conversely, certain omega-6 fatty acids found in animal-derived products can exacerbate inflammation. Incorporating omega-3-rich foods into your diet or taking supplements, typically at *doses of 1,000 mg once or twice daily*, may offer benefits for managing diverticulitis symptoms and potentially reducing the risk of colon cancer. However, individuals taking blood-thinning medications like warfarin or aspirin should exercise caution when supplementing with fish oil, as it can enhance the blood-thinning effects of these medications. Prior consultation with a healthcare provider is crucial in such cases.

For individuals experiencing constipation or diarrhea associated with diverticulitis, fiber supplements such as psyllium or methylcellulose may provide relief. These supplements work by increasing stool bulk and facilitating easier passage. However, it's important to note that initial use of fiber supplements may lead to gas and bloating. Seeking guidance from a healthcare professional before integrating fiber supplements into your regimen is advisable.

Probiotics are beneficial bacteria akin to those naturally present in the digestive system, crucial for maintaining overall health. They are available over-the-counter in various forms such as capsules, tablets, and powders, and can also *be found in certain foods like yogurt and fermented vegetables.*

Different probiotic strains exist, each with distinct characteristics. Among them, strains primarily containing Lactobacillus casei have shown promising outcomes in research studies.

Herbal remedies offer a natural approach to fortify and balance the body's systems. However, it's essential to consult with your healthcare provider before embarking on any herbal treatment regimen. Herbs can be consumed as dried extracts (capsules, powders, or teas), glycerites (extracts in glycerine), or tinctures (extracts in alcohol). For tea preparations, steep 1 teaspoon of the herb in a cup of hot water, covered, for 5 to 10 minutes for leaf or flower-based herbs, and 10 to 20 minutes for root-based herbs. Aim to consume 2 to 4 cups per day of herbal tea, or follow dosage instructions provided for tinctures.

Several herbs are commonly employed in managing gastrointestinal ailments:

Flaxseed (*Linum usitatissimum*) may aid in diverticulosis treatment by supplying fiber and serving as a bulk-forming laxative. Ground flaxseed at a dosage of 15 grams per day is recommended.

Slippery elm (*Ulmus fulva*) functions as a demulcent, safeguarding irritated tissues and fostering healing. Daily intake ranges from 60 to 320 milligrams, or alternatively, mix 1 teaspoon of powdered slippery elm with water and consume it 3 to 4 times daily.

Cat's claw (*Uncaria tomentosa*) possesses anti-inflammatory properties. However, caution should be exercised, particularly among pregnant individuals, those with autoimmune diseases, or leukemia patients, as cat's claw may interact with certain medications.

Wild yam (*Dioscorea villosa*) warrants consultation with a healthcare professional, especially for individuals with breast cancer, prostate cancer, or any hormonally-related condition. There are concerns regarding potential clot formation in individuals with Protein S deficiency.

Marshmallow (*Althaea officinalis*) acts as both a demulcent and emollient. Prepare marshmallow tea by steeping 2 to 5 grams of dried leaf or 5 grams of dried root in 1 cup of boiling water, then strain and cool. However, individuals with diabetes should exercise caution, as marshmallow may interfere with medication absorption and negatively impact lithium levels.

Chamomile (*Matricaria recutita*) can be consumed as tea, with a recommended intake of 1 to 3 cups daily.

Steep 3 grams of chamomile flower heads in 1 cup of boiling water, strain, and allow to cool. It's advisable to avoid chamomile if pregnant, taking birth control pills, or with a history of hormone-related cancers. Additionally, high doses may interact with blood-thinning medications, and individuals allergic to Ragweed or related plants should abstain from chamomile consumption.

Licorice (*Glycyrrhiza glabra***)** possesses properties that can alleviate spasms and inflammation within the gastrointestinal tract. However, it's crucial to exercise caution when using licorice, especially over an extended period or if you have underlying health conditions such as high blood pressure, heart failure, kidney disease, or hypokalemia. Opt for products containing only DGL (deglycyrrhizinated licorice), which indicates the removal of the component responsible for raising blood pressure.

Homeopathy involves the utilization of specific remedies tailored to individual constitutional types, encompassing physical, emotional, and intellectual aspects. While research on homeopathic treatments for diverticular disease remains limited, experienced practitioners may recommend remedies based on clinical experience and patient assessment.

Belladonna: Suitable for sudden abdominal pain and cramping alleviated by firm pressure, particularly effective if constipation accompanies the pain.

Bryonia: Recommended for abdominal pain aggravated by movement but relieved by heat, especially beneficial if vomiting or constipation with dry, hard stools accompanies the discomfort.

Colocynthis: Helpful for sharp, cramping abdominal pains relieved by pressure, particularly indicated if restlessness and diarrhea accompany the pain.

Acupuncture is another alternative therapy that may offer relief from pain and associated symptoms of diverticular disease. Acupuncturists tailor treatments to address individual imbalances in qi (energy) flow along meridians. Through acupuncture and Chinese medicine, efforts are made to promote overall gastrointestinal well-being.

CHAPTER III: A DEEP DIVE INTO DIVERTICULITIS NUTRITION

Studies indicate that **consuming a diet low in fiber and high in red meat might raise the likelihood of developing diverticulitis,** which involves inflammation of one or multiple pouches in the colon wall. Conversely, **incorporating high-fiber foods into your diet while reducing red meat consumption could potentially decrease this risk.**

According to the Dietary Guidelines for Americans, 2020–2025, it's recommended to consume 14 grams of dietary fiber per 1,000 calories consumed. For instance, for a 2,000-calorie daily diet, *the fiber intake suggestion is 28 grams per day.*

If you experience chronic symptoms of diverticular disease or have a history of diverticulitis, your doctor may advise increasing your intake of fiber-rich foods. They might recommend incorporating meals containing high-fiber options, such as a bowl of whole-grain cereal with fresh berries alongside high-fiber crackers and raspberries.

Consulting with a healthcare professional, like your doctor or a dietitian, can help you plan meals tailored to your specific fiber needs. They may suggest gradually increasing your fiber intake to allow your body to adjust to the dietary changes.

In the past, individuals with diverticulosis or diverticular disease were often advised to avoid certain foods like nuts, popcorn, and seeds. However, recent research suggests that these foods are not necessarily harmful to individuals with these conditions.

If you have diverticulosis or diverticular disease, it's essential to discuss potential dietary modifications with your doctor to determine if adjustments to your eating habits are necessary.

Food as Medicine: Importance of Diet in Managing Diverticulitis

Consume a high-fiber diet if you have diverticulosis, as fiber plays a crucial role in softening stool and preventing constipation. Additionally, it can help alleviate pressure in the colon and reduce the likelihood of diverticulitis flare-ups.

High-fiber foods to include in your diet are:

- Beans and legumes
- Whole grains like bran, whole wheat bread, and oatmeal
- Brown and wild rice
- Fruits such as apples, bananas, and pears
- Vegetables like broccoli, carrots, corn, and squash
- Whole wheat pasta

If you're not accustomed to a high-fiber diet, introduce fiber gradually to avoid bloating and discomfort. Aim to consume between 25 to 30 grams of fiber daily and ensure you drink at least 8 cups of fluids daily to soften stool. Regular exercise can also aid in promoting bowel movements and preventing constipation.

When your colon is not inflamed, you can tolerate popcorn, nuts, and seeds in your diet.

During diverticulitis flare-ups, adhere to a clear liquid diet as recommended by your doctor. Progress from clear liquids to low-fiber solids and then back to your regular diet as instructed by your healthcare provider.

A clear liquid diet entails avoiding solid foods and opting for liquids without pulp. During this period, you may consume:

- Broth
- Clear juices like apple, cranberry, and grape (avoid orange juice)
- Jell-O
- Popsicles

When transitioning back to solid foods during the healing process, opt for low-fiber options. These include:

- Canned or cooked fruit without seeds or skin, like applesauce and melon
- Canned or thoroughly cooked vegetables without seeds and skin
- Dairy products such as cheese, milk, and yogurt
- Eggs

- Low-fiber cereals
- Ground or tender, well-cooked meat
- Pasta
- White bread and white rice

As your symptoms improve, typically within two to four days, you can gradually reintroduce 5 to 15 grams of fiber per day into your diet. Once symptoms have subsided completely, you can resume your regular high-fiber diet.

The Nutritional Puzzle: Goals of a Diverticulitis Diet

In the treatment of diverticulitis, **the primary objective is to alleviate inflammation and allow the colon to heal**. The approach to treatment varies depending on the severity of symptoms and the patient's overall health status.

For mild cases of diverticulitis, patients may receive treatment at home. This typically involves a regimen of oral antibiotics to combat the infection, along with analgesics (pain relievers) to manage discomfort. Bed rest is often recommended to minimize strain on the colon, and a clear liquid diet is advised to provide essential hydration without taxing the digestive system.

However, for individuals with *more severe symptoms or complications, hospitalization becomes necessary.* In a hospital setting, patients can receive more intensive care, including intravenous antibiotics for faster and more effective treatment. Close monitoring by healthcare professionals ensures prompt intervention if complications arise.

In cases where diverticulitis recurs frequently or leads to complications such as abscess formation, bowel perforation, or fistula formation, surgical intervention may be warranted. Surgery aims to address the underlying issue by removing the affected portion of the colon. This procedure, known as **resection**, may involve reconnecting the healthy segments of the colon (primary anastomosis) if feasible. However, if the condition of the colon is compromised, a temporary diverting colostomy may be created. This diversion allows stool to bypass the affected area while the colon heals. Once the inflammation resolves and the colon regains its strength, the colostomy can be reversed through a subsequent surgical procedure, restoring the natural flow of waste through the digestive system.

Overall, the treatment approach for diverticulitis is tailored to each individual's specific needs, with the goal of alleviating symptoms, preventing complications, and promoting long-term gastrointestinal health.

Why Your Diet Matters More Than You Think: Benefits of a Well-Planned Diet

In the effort to manage diverticulitis, meal planning plays a crucial role and is a simple yet effective step toward achieving your health goals. There are numerous benefits to planning your meals in advance, all of which contribute to improving your overall well-being.

Consider these advantages of meal planning:

1. Control Portion Sizes:

By planning your meals, you gain insight into the portion sizes you're consuming. This helps prevent overeating, particularly when dining out, where servings tend to be larger than necessary.

2. Promote Healthy Eating:

When hunger strikes and blood sugar levels dip, it's easy to grab whatever food is most convenient, often opting for unhealthy choices like fast food. Meal planning circumvents this issue by ensuring you have balanced meals readily available, packed with nutritious foods that are prepped and ready to eat.

Unhealthy food choices are often made due to convenience. However, if we take the time to plan meals, create a grocery list, and have fruits, vegetables, whole grains, and beans on hand, they become convenient options that are more likely to be consumed.

3. **Save Time:**

Feeling hungry and realizing you haven't planned anything can be pretty stressful. Instead of staring into your fridge or pantry, wondering what to cook, meal planning ensures your healthy meal is ready in minutes. Plus, it saves you the hassle of cleaning up afterward.

4. Save Money:

Who doesn't love saving a few bucks? Meal planning is a smart way to do just that. Not only do you cut down on restaurant expenses, but buying items in bulk, a part of meal planning, can also significantly reduce costs. Plus, sticking to your grocery list helps avoid those impulse purchases that can add up.

5. Avoid Wasting Food:

With meal planning, you hit the grocery store with a game plan, knowing exactly how every item will be used. When each ingredient serves a purpose, you won't find yourself tossing out forgotten items from the back of your fridge.

Whether you're cooking for a crowd or just yourself, investing a bit of time each week to plan your meals pays off. The key is to carve out a little time in your schedule to make it happen.

CHAPTER IV: MAKING SENSE OF FOOD CHOICES

In certain situations, your doctor may recommend specific dietary adjustments to manage diverticulitis more effectively and reduce the risk of worsening symptoms over time. During an acute diverticulitis episode, your doctor might advise following either a low-fiber diet or a clear liquid diet to alleviate your symptoms.

As symptoms improve, they may suggest maintaining a low-fiber diet until symptoms fully resolve, gradually transitioning to a high-fiber diet to prevent future flare-ups.

Low-fiber food options suitable for diverticulitis symptoms may include:

- Refined grains like white rice, white bread, or white pasta (if you're gluten intolerant, avoid gluten-containing foods)
- Dry, low-fiber cereals
- Processed fruits such as applesauce or canned peaches
- Cooked animal proteins like fish, poultry, or eggs
- Healthy oils like olive oil
- Vegetables like yellow squash, zucchini, or pumpkin without skin or seeds, as well as cooked spinach, beets, carrots, or asparagus
- Potatoes without skin
- Fruit and vegetable juices

In some cases, your doctor may prescribe a clear liquid diet as a more restrictive measure to alleviate diverticulitis symptoms. This diet is typically recommended for a short duration.

A clear liquid diet typically includes:

- Water
- Ice chips
- Clear soup broth or stock
- Gelatin, like Jell-O
- Tea or coffee without additives
- Clear electrolyte drinks

Regardless of whether you're on a clear liquid diet or not, **it's important to maintain proper hydration by**

drinking plenty of water daily to support gastrointestinal health.

Consult with your doctor before making significant dietary changes.

After recovery from a clear liquid diet, your doctor might advise gradually reintroducing low-fiber foods into your diet, eventually transitioning to a high-fiber diet.

Regarding foods to avoid during diverticulitis, there's a shift in expert opinions. While doctors previously recommended a low-fiber, clear liquid diet during flare-ups, some experts now question the necessity of avoiding specific foods for diverticulosis or diverticulitis. However, management varies by individual, and some may find avoiding certain foods beneficial.

In cases of mild flare-ups, some doctors still recommend a clear liquid diet initially. As symptoms improve, they may advise transitioning to a low fiber diet until symptoms subside, followed by gradually increasing fiber intake to a high fiber diet.

High FODMAP foods

Adopting a low FODMAP diet can offer benefits to individuals dealing with irritable bowel syndrome (IBS) and might also aid some people managing diverticulitis.

FODMAPs represent various types of carbohydrates, standing for **fermentable oligosaccharides, disaccharides, monosaccharides, and polyols.**

Some studies propose that adhering to a low FODMAP diet might mitigate colon pressure, potentially assisting in diverticulitis prevention or management.

On this diet, individuals steer clear of high FODMAP foods, including items such as:

- Certain fruits like apples, pears, and plums
- Dairy products such as milk, yogurt, and ice cream
- Fermented foods like sauerkraut or kimchi
- Beans and legumes
- Foods rich in trans fats
- Soy

- Cabbage
- Brussels sprouts
- Onions and garlic

Red and processed meats

Research from 2018 indicates that a diet rich in red and processed meats might elevate the risk of diverticulitis development, while a diet abundant in fruits, vegetables, and whole grains could lower this risk.

High-sugar and high-fat foods

The conventional Western diet often teems with fat and sugar but lacks fiber, potentially heightening the likelihood of diverticulitis. A study from 2017, encompassing over 46,000 male participants, suggests that steering clear of the following foods might aid in diverticulitis prevention or symptom reduction:

- Red meat
- Refined grains
- Full-fat dairy
- Fried foods

High-Fiber Foods: Your Gut's Greatest Allies

In the past, experts referred to fiber as a type of carbohydrate that the body couldn't digest. However, recent scientific discoveries have blurred the lines, as some digestible substances share properties with fiber, making its definition more complex.

Scientists classify fiber in various ways:

Dietary fiber: Naturally found in plants we consume.

Added fiber: Fiber incorporated by manufacturers into certain products to enhance their health benefits.

Soluble fibers: These dissolve in water and are digestible.

Insoluble fibers: These cannot be digested.

Detailed explanations of these fiber types are provided in the section "*Fiber: The Foundation of a Diverticulitis Diet*" of this cookbook.

Some examples of healthy high-fiber foods:

Pears (3.1 grams): Besides being tasty and nutritious, pears can satisfy sweet cravings while providing a good source of fiber. They contain about 5.5 grams of fiber in a medium-sized, raw pear or 3.1 grams per 100 grams.

Strawberries (2 grams): Delicious and healthy, strawberries are perfect for enjoying fresh as a summer dessert or snack. Alongside fiber, they offer vitamin C, manganese, and various antioxidants. A cup of fresh strawberries contains about 3 grams of fiber, or 2 grams per 100 grams.

Avocado (6.7 grams): High in healthy fats, avocados are rich in fiber and provide essential nutrients like vitamin C, potassium, magnesium, vitamin E, and various B vitamins. A cup of raw avocado yields approximately 10 grams of fiber, or 6.7 grams per 100 grams.

Oats (10.1 grams): Oats stand out as an exceptional fiber source packed with vitamins, minerals, and antioxidants. They feature beta-glucan, a potent soluble fiber that may assist in managing blood sugar and cholesterol levels. A cup of raw oats contains about 16.5 grams of fiber, or 10.1 grams per 100 grams.

Apples (2.4 grams): Apples are not just delicious but also satisfying, offering both soluble and insoluble fiber when consumed whole. A medium-sized raw apple provides around 4.4 grams of fiber, or 2.4 grams per 100 grams.

Raspberries (6.5 grams): Known for their distinctive flavor, raspberries are a nutritious fruit rich in fiber, vitamin C, and manganese. A cup of raw raspberries supplies approximately 8 grams of fiber, or 6.5 grams per 100 grams.

Other high-fiber berries: Including berries in your diet adds not just sweetness but also fiber to desserts, oatmeal, and smoothies, or as a healthy snack option during the day. Blueberries offer 2.4 grams of fiber per 100-gram serving, while blackberries provide 5.3 grams.

Bananas (2.6 grams): Bananas are a nutrient-rich fruit containing vitamin C, vitamin B6, and potassium. Additionally, green or unripe bananas are rich in resistant starch, an indigestible carbohydrate similar to fiber. A medium-sized banana contains about 3.1 grams of fiber, or 2.6 grams per 100 grams.

Carrots (2.8 grams): Carrots, whether enjoyed raw or cooked, are versatile root vegetables. Alongside fiber, they offer a range of nutrients including vitamin K, vitamin B6, magnesium, and beta carotene, which converts into vitamin A in the body. A cup of raw carrots contains about 3.6 grams of fiber, or 2.8 grams per 100 grams.

Beets (2 grams): Beets, also known as beetroot, are nutrient-rich root vegetables packed with folate, iron, copper, manganese, and potassium. They're also a source of inorganic nitrates, which have potential benefits for regulating blood pressure and improving exercise performance. A cup of raw beets provides approximately 3.8 grams of fiber, or 2 grams per 100 grams.

Broccoli (2.6 grams): Broccoli belongs to the cruciferous vegetable family, known for its dense nutrient profile. Rich in fiber, broccoli also delivers vitamin C, vitamin K, folate, B vitamins, potassium, iron, and manganese. It contains antioxidants and compounds that may aid in cancer prevention. With relatively high protein content compared to other vegetables, broccoli offers 2.4 grams of fiber per cup, or 2.6 grams per 100 grams.

Artichoke (5.4 grams): Artichokes are nutrient powerhouses, boasting a variety of essential vitamins and minerals along with a significant fiber content. One raw globe or French artichoke provides around 6.9 grams of fiber, or 5.4 grams per 100 grams.

Brussels sprouts (3.8 grams): Brussels sprouts, akin to broccoli, belong to the cruciferous vegetable family. Packed with fiber, they're also abundant in vitamin K, potassium, folate, and potentially beneficial antioxidants. Raw Brussels sprouts offer around 3.3 grams of fiber per cup, or 3.8 grams per 100 grams.

Other vegetables rich in fiber include kale with 4.1 grams, spinach with 2.2 grams, and tomatoes with 1.2 grams.

Lentils (10.7 grams): Lentils are a budget-friendly, adaptable, and highly nutritious legume. They're prized for their fiber, protein, and diverse nutrient profile. Cooked lentils contain approximately 13.1 grams of fiber per cup, or 10.7 grams per 100 grams.

Kidney Beans (7.4 grams): Kidney beans, a common legume variety, offer plant-based protein and various nutrients. They provide about 12.2 grams of fiber per cup when cooked, or 7.4 grams per 100 grams.

Split Peas (8.3 grams): Split peas are derived from dried, split, and peeled pea seeds. Often found in split pea soup and other dishes, they're notable for their high fiber content, offering around 16.3 grams per cup when cooked, or 8.3 grams per 100 grams.

Chickpeas (7 grams): Chickpeas, also known as garbanzo beans, are legumes renowned for their fiber, protein, and mineral content. Commonly used in hummus, curries, and salads, they provide approximately 12.5 grams of fiber per cooked cup, or 7.6 grams per 100 grams.

Other high-fiber legumes are abundant in protein, fiber, and essential nutrients, offering a delicious and cost-effective nutritional option when prepared thoughtfully. Some of these legumes include:

Cooked Black Beans: Providing 8.7 grams of fiber per serving.

Cooked Edamame: Offering 5.2 grams of fiber.

Cooked Lima Beans: With 7 grams of fiber.

Baked Beans: Contributing 5.5 grams of fiber.

Quinoa (2.8 grams): Quinoa, a pseudo-cereal, stands as a fiber-rich and protein-packed choice, particularly beneficial for plant-based diets. It boasts additional nutrients such as magnesium, iron, zinc, potassium, and antioxidants. A cup of cooked quinoa contains 5.2 grams of fiber, or 2.8 grams per 100 grams.

Popcorn (14.5 grams): Popcorn can be a delightful and fiber-rich snack option. When air-popped, it boasts a high fiber content per calorie. However, the addition of fats or sugars diminishes the fiber-to-calorie ratio.

Air-popped popcorn contains 1.15 grams of fiber per cup or 14.5 grams per 100 grams.

Almonds (13.3 grams): Almonds are not only rich in fiber but also provide healthy fats, vitamin E, manganese, and magnesium. They can be ground into almond flour for baking, making them a versatile and nutritious option. Three tablespoons of almonds offer 4 grams of fiber, or 13.3 grams per 100 grams.

Chia Seeds (34.4 grams): Chia seeds, despite their small size, pack a powerful nutritional punch. These tiny black seeds are rich in fiber and boast high levels of magnesium, phosphorus, and calcium.

You can add chia seeds into your diet by mixing them into jam or adding them to homemade granola bars.

With 9.75 grams of fiber per ounce of dried chia seeds, or 34.4 grams per 100 grams, they stand as an exceptional fiber source.

Other nuts and seeds also offer significant fiber content, such as:

Fresh Coconut: Providing 9 grams of fiber.

Pistachios: Offering 10.6 grams of fiber.

Walnuts: Contributing 6.7 grams of fiber.

Sunflower Seeds: Providing 8.6 grams of fiber.

Pumpkin Seeds: Containing 6 grams of fiber.

NOTE: All values are based on a 100-gram portion.

Sweet Potatoes (3 grams): Sweet potatoes, a beloved tuber known for its sweet flavor and satisfying nature, are rich in beta carotene, B vitamins, and various minerals.

They can serve as a delectable bread substitute or form the foundation for nachos. With a medium-sized boiled sweet potato (without skin) containing 3.8 grams of fiber, or 3 grams per 100 grams, they offer both flavor and fiber.

Dark Chocolate (10.9 grams): Dark chocolate, when consumed in moderation and with high cocoa content, can be a source of essential nutrients and antioxidants.

Opt for dark chocolate with a cocoa content of 70%–95% or higher to reap its benefits, while avoiding products with excessive added sugar. With 3.1 grams of fiber in a 1-ounce piece of 70%–85% cacao, or 10.9

grams per 100 grams, dark chocolate can be a delightful and nutritious treat.

Low-Fiber Fare: Foods to Limit or Avoid

Low-fiber protein sources include meat, fish, poultry, tofu, and various nut products. Opt for tender cuts of meat or ground meat for easier digestion. Tofu and fish, including shellfish, are also gentle on the digestive system. Smooth peanut butter and eggs are additional options within this category.

When it comes to dairy, choose low-fiber options such as milk and cheese. This includes milk variations like chocolate milk, buttermilk, and milk drinks. Opt for yogurt without seeds or granola, sour cream, cheese, cottage cheese, and custard or pudding. Ice cream or frozen desserts without nuts are also suitable.

For bread, cereals, and grains, opt for low-fiber varieties such as white bread, waffles, French toast, plain white rolls, or toasted white bread. Pretzels, plain pasta or noodles, white rice, and crackers like zwieback, melba, and matzoh are good choices. Choose cereals without whole grains, added fiber, seeds, raisins, or other dried fruit.

Include low-fiber vegetables and potatoes into your diet. Choose tender, well-cooked fresh or canned vegetables without seeds, stems, or skins. Cooked sweet or white potatoes without skins are also gentle on the digestive system. Additionally, strained vegetable juices without pulp or spices can be included.

Low-fiber options for fruits and desserts include soft canned or cooked fruit without seeds or skins, consumed in small amounts. You can also enjoy small portions of well-ripened bananas, strained or clear juices, and soft cantaloupe or honeydew melon.

When it comes to desserts, opt for cookies and other treats without whole grains, dried fruit, berries, nuts, or coconut. Sherbet and popsicles are refreshing options to consider.

In addition, there are several other low-fiber foods to include in your diet. These include mayonnaise and mild salad dressings, margarine, butter, cream, and oils in small amounts. Plain gravies, bouillon, and broth are suitable choices. Mild condiments like ketchup and mustard can be added for flavor. You can also use spices, cooked herbs, and salt to enhance taste. For sweetness, opt for sugar, honey, and syrup. Clear jellies, hard candy, marshmallows, and plain chocolate are also low-fiber indulgences.

Extra One Week Meal Plan

This example menu offers a range of meals that are rich in nutrients, fiber, and protein, aiming to support your weight loss objectives.

It's important to tailor the portions according to your personal requirements. Additionally, while snack suggestions are provided, they are entirely optional.

Monday

Breakfast: overnight oats made with rolled oats, chia seeds, and milk, topped with fresh berries and pumpkin seeds

Lunch: premade egg-and-veggie muffins with a fresh basil-and-tomato salad and some avocado

Snack: mango-spinach smoothie

Dinner: homemade cauliflower-crust pizza topped with pesto, mushrooms, peppers, a handful of spinach, and marinated chicken or tempeh

Tuesday

Breakfast: breakfast smoothie made with kale, frozen cherries, banana, protein powder, flax seeds, and milk

Lunch: mixed green salad with cucumber, bell pepper, tomato, corn, sweet potato, olives, and grilled salmon or roasted chickpeas

Snack: sliced apple with peanut butter

Dinner: red lentil dahl served on a bed of baby spinach and brown rice

Wednesday

Breakfast: Spanish omelet made with eggs, potatoes, onions, and peppers, served with a side of salsa

Lunch: leftover red lentil dahl and fresh spinach over brown rice

Snack: homemade trail mix using your favorite unsalted, unroasted nuts and unsweetened dried fruit

Dinner: chicken or tofu meatballs in a marinara sauce served with spaghetti squash on a bed of mixed baby greens and topped with Parmesan cheese or nutritional yeast

Thursday

Breakfast: yogurt topped with fresh fruit and chopped walnuts

Lunch: kale salad topped with a poached egg or marinated seitan, as well as dried cranberries, cherry tomatoes, whole-grain pita chips, and an avocado-mango dressing

Snack: carrots, radishes, and cherry tomatoes dipped in hummus

Dinner: beef or black-bean burger topped with lettuce, tomato, roasted peppers, caramelized onions, and pickles, served on a small whole-wheat bun and peppers and onions on the side

Friday

Breakfast: breakfast salad made with spinach, homemade granola, walnuts, blueberries, coconut flakes, and a raspberry vinaigrette, as well as 1–2 hard-boiled eggs for extra protein if you like

Lunch: homemade veggie spring rolls, dipped in peanut butter sauce and served with a side of raw veggies

Snack: whole-wheat crackers with cheese or a spicy mashed black bean spread

Dinner: chili served on a bed of greens and wild rice

Saturday

Breakfast: pumpkin pancakes topped with Greek or plant-based yogurt, chopped nuts, and fresh strawberries

Lunch: leftover chili served on a bed of greens and wild rice

Snack: nut-and-dried-fruit trail mix

Dinner: shrimp or bean fajitas with grilled onions, bell peppers, and guacamole, served on a corn tortilla

Sunday

Breakfast: overnight oats topped with chopped pecans, mango, and coconut flakes

Lunch: tuna or chickpea salad, served atop mixed greens with sliced avocado, sliced apple, and walnuts

Snack: yogurt with fruit

Dinner: grilled salmon or tempeh, potatoes, and sautéed kale

Ideas for dietary restrictions

Generally speaking, meat, fish, eggs, and dairy can be replaced by plant-based alternatives, such as tofu, tempeh, seitan, beans, flax or chia seeds, as well as plant-based milk and yogurts.

Gluten-containing grains and flours can be substituted for quinoa, millet, oats, buckwheat, amaranth, teff, corn, and sorghum.

Carb-rich grains and starchy vegetables can be replaced by lower-carb alternatives.

For instance, try spiralized noodles or spaghetti squash instead of pasta, cauliflower rice instead of couscous or rice, lettuce leaves instead of taco shells, and seaweed or rice paper instead of tortilla wraps.

Just keep in mind that completely excluding a food group may require you to take supplements to meet your daily nutrient needs.

Grocery Guides: Stocking Your Pantry with Success

Next time you're at the grocery store, make sure to pick up these items. They're excellent sources of fiber, which not only lowers your LDL ("bad") cholesterol but also promotes gut health and digestion, while keeping you feeling full.

Fruits and Vegetables:

Apples, bananas, oranges, and strawberries: These fruits each offer about 3 to 4 grams of fiber, with the apple peel being the richest source.

Raspberries: Leading the fiber pack with 8 grams per cup.

Mangoes, persimmons, and guavas: A mango supplies 5 grams, a persimmon provides 6 grams, and a cup of guava offers roughly 9 grams of fiber.

Dark-colored vegetables: Carrots, beets, broccoli, collard greens, and Swiss chard are fiber-rich choices.

Artichokes stand out with an impressive 10 grams of fiber in a medium-sized one.

Potatoes: Whether Russet, red, or sweet, these spuds deliver at least 3 grams of fiber each when eaten with the skin.

Dry and Canned Goods:

Beans: Navy and white beans top the list for fiber content, but all varieties—black, garbanzo, kidney, lima, or pinto—are fiber-packed. These versatile legumes are perfect for soups, chilis, salads, and serve as a protein-rich alternative to red meat.

Other legumes: Peas, soybeans (edamame), and lentils are additional fiber-rich options.

Bread and Grains:

Cereal: Opt for cereals boasting 5 or more grams of fiber per serving for a substantial fiber boost.

Whole-grain breads: Choose varieties like seven-grain, dark rye, cracked wheat, or pumpernickel for added fiber.

Whole grains: Experiment with bulgur wheat, brown rice, wild rice, or barley as nutritious alternatives to white rice.

The Snack Aisle

Nuts and seeds are excellent sources of fiber. For instance, an ounce of sunflower seeds, pumpkin seeds, pistachios, or almonds provides you with at least 3 grams of fiber. However, keep in mind that they are calorie-dense, so it's best to enjoy them in moderation.

Popcorn is another great option. Three cups of air-popped popcorn contain about 4 grams of fiber.

The Cold Case

Consider trying foods with added fiber. While milk, dairy products, and most juices naturally contain little to no fiber, there are new products emerging with added fiber. Keep an eye out for labels on orange juice, milk, and yogurt indicating that fiber has been added or that they are "fiber fortified."

Meal Planning Resources: Practical Tools for Meal Planning

Utilize these resources to streamline your meal planning and grocery shopping endeavors while maintaining a healthy diet on a budget.

- Nutrition on a Budget
- Local Food Directories: National Farmers Market Directory
- MyPlate Tip Sheets
- Healthy, Thrifty Holiday Menus
- Seasonal Produce Guide
- Food Shopping Tips
- Heart-Healthy Foods: Shopping List
- Sample 7-Day Meal Plan
- Smart Shopping: Shop with Meals in Mind
- Weekly Meal Planner

- Modifying a Recipe to Be Healthier
- Mediterranean Eating on a Budget
- Shop Smart
- Weekly Menu Planner
- Meal Planning
- The Essential Guide to Meal Prep for College Students
- How to Make a Meal Plan

CHAPTER V: HEALTHY DIVERTICULITIS-FRIENDLY RECIPES

DIVERTICULITIS-FRIENDLY CLEAR LIQUID DIET

Lemon Ginger Herbal Tea

Ingredients

1 cup water

1 inch fresh ginger root, peeled

1 teaspoon lemon juice

Instructions

Boil the water, then add the sliced ginger root.

Allow it to simmer for about 10 minutes, strain, add lemon juice and drink warm.

Chicken Broth Soup

Ingredients

2 chicken breasts

2 liters water

Salt, to taste

Instructions

Boil the chicken breasts in water until fully cooked.

Remove the chicken (save for later use if wanted), strain the broth and add salt to taste.

Apple Juice Jelly

Ingredients

2 cups clear apple juice

1 packet unflavored gelatin

Instructions

Heat 1 cup of apple juice until it begins to boil.

Sprinkle the gelatin over 1 cup of cold apple juice and allow it to dissolve.

Add the hot apple juice and stir until the gelatin is fully dissolved.

Chill until set.

Clear Veggie Broth

Ingredients

2 liters water

1 onion

2 carrots

2 celery sticks

Instructions

Chop the vegetables and boil in water for about 45 minutes.

Strain the broth and discard the vegetables.

Refreshing Grape Juice Slushie

Ingredients

2 cups clear grape juice

Ice cubes

Instructions

Pour the grape juice into a blender, add ice cubes, and blend until it reaches a slushie consistency.

Herbal Peppermint Tea

Ingredients

1 peppermint tea bag

1 cup boiling water

Instructions

Place the tea bag in a cup and pour boiling water over it. Steep for 3-5 minutes, remove the tea bag, and enjoy.

Clear Vegetable Soup

Ingredients

2 liters water

1 leek

2 garlic cloves

Salt, to taste

Instructions

Chop the leek and garlic, add them to boiling water and cook for about 45 minutes. Strain the broth, add salt to taste, and serve.

Pineapple Juice Jelly

Ingredients

2 cups clear pineapple juice

1 packet unflavored gelatin

Instructions

Heat 1 cup of pineapple juice until it begins to boil.

Sprinkle the gelatin over 1 cup of cold pineapple juice and allow it to dissolve.

Add the hot pineapple juice and stir until the gelatin is fully dissolved.

Chill until set.

Green Tea with Honey

Ingredients

1 green tea bag

1 cup boiling water

1 teaspoon honey

Instructions

Steep the green tea bag in boiling water for 3 minutes.

Remove the tea bag, add honey, stir, and enjoy.

Watermelon Juice Slushie

Ingredients

2 cups clear watermelon juice

Ice cubes

Instructions

Pour the watermelon juice into a blender, add ice cubes, and blend until it reaches a slushie consistency.

Clear Chicken Broth

Ingredients

Chicken broth as required (low sodium)

Salt to taste

Instructions

In a small pot, heat the chicken broth over medium heat until it comes to a gentle boil.

Add salt to taste, if desired.

Simmer for a few minutes to enhance the flavors.

Remove.

Clear Vegetable Broth

Ingredients

Vegetable broth as required

Salt, and pepper to taste

Instructions

The vegetable broth should be heated in a small saucepan over medium heat until it just begins to simmer.

Salt to taste, if you'd like.

Simmer for a while.

Take the broth off the heat.

Serve hot.

DIVERTICULITIS-FRIENDLY HIGH FIBER SOUPS

Slow Cooker Lentil, Sausage and Kale Soup

Ingredients

2 Tablespoons olive oil

1 Pound Italian seasoned turkey sausage, casings removed

1 onion, chopped

2 carrots, chopped

2 celery stalks, chopped

1 Teaspoon Italian seasoning

1/2 Teaspoon black pepper

2 garlic cloves, chopped

15 Ounces diced tomatoes

1 1/2 Cup green or brown lentils

4 Cups vegetable or chicken broth

3 Cups kale, chopped roughly

Instructions

In a slow cooker, heat the olive oil and brown/sear the Italian turkey sausage, crumbling with a wooden spoon.

Add onions, carrots, celery, and Italian seasoning and pepper, and cook until vegetables soften about 5-7 minutes. Add garlic and cook another minute.

Add tomatoes, lentils, and broth and stir to combine all ingredients.

Cook covered on low for 6-8 hours, until lentils get tender, not mushy.

Add kale and stir and cook until kale wilts. Adjust seasoning.

Serve with grated Parmesan on top if desired and crusty whole-wheat bread.

Note- If the slow cooker does not have a sear/browning function, the sausage and vegetables and seasonings can be cooked in a separate skillet and then added to the slow cooker.

Smooth Broccoli Soup

Ingredients

2 Tablespoons olive oil

1 leek, chopped

1 celery stalk, chopped

2 garlic cloves, minced

3 small potatoes, unpeeled, chopped

1/2 Teaspoon salt

1 bay leaf

3 Cups vegetable broth

1 1/2 Cup broccoli florets

Instructions

In a large soup pan, heat oil over medium-high heat. Cook leek, celery, garlic, potatoes, salt and bay leaf until lightly browned.

Add stock and bring to a boil. Reduce heat, cover and simmer 30 minutes.

Add broccoli florets to pot and bring back to a boil. Reduce heat, cover, and simmer another 15 minutes or until all vegetables are tender.

Remove from heat and let cool. Remove bay leaf. Puree soup with a hand blender, until smooth. Serve.

Pea and Pesto Soup

Ingredients

1 Cup yellow split peas, uncooked, rinsed

2 Cups chicken broth

2 1/2 Cups water

2 Tablespoons pesto, homemade or store bought

1 small zucchini, seeded and sliced

1/2 Cup green onions, chopped

Instructions

In a large soup pot, combine split peas, broth and water and bring to a boil.

Reduce heat, cover, and simmer for 20 minutes.

Stir in pesto, zucchini, and green onions; simmer for 15 to 20 more minutes. Garnish with Parmesan cheese, if desired.

Creamy Carrot Soup

Ingredients

Olive oil

Chopped carrots

Chopped onions

Minced garlic cloves

Curry powder (optional)

Chicken broth

Carrot juice

Instructions

In a large soup pot, heat oil over medium heat.

Add carrots and onion and continue to cook for about 6-8 minutes. Add garlic and curry powder and cook for another minute.

Next, add broth and 1/2 tsp salt and simmer over low heat. Cover and let simmer for about 15 minutes.

Add carrot juice and mix well. Pour the soup into a blender. Return the soup to the pan and season with salt and pepper. Serve.

Creamy Carrot Soup

Ingredients

Boneless, skinless chicken breast, thinly sliced as per requirement

1 red bell pepper, sliced

1 zucchini, sliced

1 carrot, sliced

2 cloves of garlic, minced

2 tablespoons low-sodium soy sauce

1 tablespoon olive oil

Salt and pepper to taste

Instructions

Heat the olive oil in a large skillet or wok over medium-high heat.

Add the minced garlic and cook for about 1 minute until fragrant.

Add the chicken slices to the skillet and stir-fry until cooked through.

Add the sliced red bell pepper, zucchini, and carrot to the skillet and continue stir-frying for about 5-7 minutes until the vegetables are tender-crisp.

Drizzle the soy sauce over the chicken and vegetables, and season with salt and pepper to taste.

Cook for another minute, stirring to combine all the flavors.

Serve the chicken and vegetable stir-fry hot with a side of cooked white rice or quinoa.

Mushroom and Ginger Soup

Ingredients

2 Teaspoons vegetable oil

3 garlic cloves, crushed

1 Tablespoon fresh ginger, grated

4 Ounces white mushrooms, sliced

4 Cups vegetable broth

1 Teaspoon low sodium soy sauce

4 Ounces bean sprouts

4 Ounces whole wheat thin pasta

4 Tablespoons fresh cilantro

Instructions

Bring a large pot of salted water to a boil.

Add pasta and cook according to package instructions until al dente. Drain.

In a large soup pot, heat oil over medium-high heat. Add garlic, ginger and mushrooms. Stir until softened, about 3-4 minutes.

Add vegetable stock and bring to boil. Add soy sauce and bean sprouts and continue to cook until tender.

To serve, place cooked noodles in individual bowls and ladle soup on top. Garnish with fresh cilantro

Kidney Bean Soup

Ingredients

3 slices bacon

1 Teaspoon garlic cloves, minced

2 shallots, chopped

1 carrots, chopped

28 Ounces kidney beans, drained

1/2 Cup quick cooking brown rice

4 Cups beef broth

2 bay leaves

1/4 Teaspoon dried basil

Instructions

In a large soup pot, cook bacon over medium heat until crisp. Crumble and set aside.

In the same pan with the bacon oil, cook garlic, shallots and carrots until tender, about 5 minutes.

Place the beans in blender and puree until smooth. Stir into the vegetable mixture in the pan.

Add the bacon, rice, broth, bay leaves and basil. Stir soup and bring pot to a boil.

Reduce heat and simmer covered, until rice is tender, 20 minutes. Serve.

Creamy Squash Soup

Ingredients

1 acorn squash, cut lengthwise, seeds removed

1 sweet potato, cut lengthwise

4 shallots, cut lengthwise

2 Tablespoons olive oil

4 garlic cloves, whole

4 Cups vegetable broth

14 Ounces cannellini beans, drained and rinsed

1/4 Cup sour cream

Instructions

Preheat oven to 375 degrees.

Brush cut sides of squash, sweet potato and shallots with oil. Place vegetables, cut side down, in a shallow roasting pan and add garlic cloves. Roast in oven until tender, about 30 – 40 minutes.

Allow vegetables to cool, and scoop out flesh of squash, sweet potato. In a soup pot, place flesh of roasted vegetables, shallots and garlic.

Add broth and bring to a boil. Reduce heat, and simmer, covered for 30 minutes, stirring occasionally.

Pour half of the beans into the soup pot and allow soup to cool. Puree soup with a hand blender, until smooth.

Add other half of beans and cream. Season to taste and simmer until warmed through, about 5 minutes. Serve.

Creamy Chickpea Soup

Ingredients

2 1/2 Cups vegetable broth

2 Cups fresh baby spinach

2 Cups tomatoes, seeded and chopped

2 Cups hummus, homemade or store bought

1 Tablespoon lemon juice

Instructions

In a medium pot, bring vegetable broth to a boil.

Add spinach and tomatoes and cook until spinach wilts, about 4 – 5 minutes.

Lower heat and stir in the hummus and lemon juice and cook until heated through.

Cannellini and Butter Bean Soup

Ingredients

1 Tablespoon olive oil

3 slices pancetta, chopped

3 garlic cloves, minced

2 medium onions, chopped

28 Ounces cannellini beans, drained and rinsed

28 Ounces butter (Lima) beans, drained and rinsed

2 Teaspoons thyme, fresh, chopped

1 Tablespoon balsamic vinegar

6 Cups vegetable stock

Instructions

In a large soup pot, heat olive oil over medium-high heat. Cook pancetta until crisp.

Add garlic and onions. Cook until onions are tender, about 5 minutes.

Stir in beans, thyme, vinegar and vegetable stock. Bring pot to a boil, reduce heat and simmer uncovered for 25 minutes. Serve.

Beef and Vegetable Soup

Ingredients

1/2 Pound stew beef, diced

1/2 bag frozen vegetable medley

1/4 Cup barley

32 Ounces beef broth

2 tomatoes, seeded and chopped

1 Teaspoon garlic powder

1 Teaspoon paprika

1 Teaspoon oregano

1 bay leaf

1 yellow or red potato, chopped

Instructions

In a large soup pot, over medium-high heat, brown ground beef.

Add frozen vegetables, barley, broth, tomatoes, garlic powder, paprika, oregano and bay leaf. Bring the pot to a boil, Reduce heat, cover and simmer for 15 minutes.

Add the potatoes and allow to simmer again for another 20 minutes or until they are tender.

Beans with Greens Soup

Ingredients

2 Tablespoons olive oil

1 onion, chopped

4 garlic cloves, minced

2 celery stalks, sliced finely

2 carrots, sliced

6 Cups chicken broth

1/4 Teaspoon thyme

1/4 Teaspoon rosemary

1 bay leaf

14 Ounces cannellini beans, drained and rinsed

1/2 Teaspoon salt

1 Cup leafy greens (kale, spinach or chard), chopped

Instructions

In a large soup pot, heat olive oil over medium heat. Add onions and cook until softened, about 3 minutes. Stir in onion, garlic, celery, and carrots and continue to cook for 5 minutes, stirring occasionally.

Add chicken broth, thyme, rosemary, and bay leaf and cook until it comes to a boil. Reduce heat and cover and simmer gently for about 45-60 minutes.

Add beans and season with salt. Add leafy greens and cook until tender, approximately 5-10 minutes, depending on the greens being used. Serve.

For a creamier texture, prior to adding the greens, the broth and vegetables can be blended with an immersion blender until desired consistency is reached.

Vegetable and Lentil Stew

Ingredients

1 Tablespoon Olive Oil

1 Diced onion

2 Cloves of minced garlic

2 Cups Diced mixed vegetables (carrots, potatoes, and green beans)

1 Cup Green or brown lentils

2 Cups Vegetable broth

1 Teaspoon Dried thyme

1/2 Teaspoon Dried rosemary

1/4 Teaspoon Salt

1/4 Teaspoon Black pepper

1/4 Cup chopped fresh parsley

Instructions

In a large pot, heat the olive oil over medium-high heat. Add the onion, garlic, mixed vegetables, and lentils. Cook for 3-4 minutes, or until the vegetables are tender.

Stir in the vegetable broth, thyme, rosemary, salt, and black pepper. Bring to a boil.

Reduce the heat to low, cover, and simmer for 20-25 minutes, or until the lentils are tender.

Stir in the parsley, and serve hot with a side of whole grain bread or crackers.

DIVERTICULITIS-FRIENDLY SALAD RECIPES

Asian Chicken Salad

Ingredients

1 Cup romaine lettuce, chopped

1 carrot, shredded

1 celery, sliced thinly

1/4 Cup red bell pepper, seeded, sliced thinly

1/2 Cup chicken breast, cut into strips

1/4 Cup mangoes

2 Tablespoons lime and ginger dressing, store bought

Instructions

In a medium bowl, toss together all ingredients until combined.

Serve alone or with whole wheat bread slices.

Tuna Cakes and Smashed Potatoes

Ingredients

Potatoes, unpeeled, chopped

2 Teaspoons salt

1/2 Cup milk

3 Tablespoons butter

3 Tablespoons canola oil

12 Ounces tuna fish, drained

Egg, beaten

2 Tablespoons green onions, diced

1/4 Cup mayonnaise

1/2 Cup whole wheat bread, cut into small pieces

Lemon juice, optional

Instructions

Cook potatoes in a small saucepan until tender. Drain. Place potatoes back in pan. Heat the milk and butter in microwave until hot. With a potato masher, roughly smash the potatoes while adding hot liquid until combined and set aside.

In a bowl, combine tuna, egg, green onions, mayonnaise, bread crumbs, and lemon juice. Form into patties. Allow to refrigerate and become firm for 10 minutes.

Heat oil over medium-high heat, cook patties until golden brown, about 2 minutes on each side. Serve with potatoes.

Bean and Couscous Salad

Ingredients

1 Cup couscous

1 1/2 Cup boiling water

1 Cup yellow bell peppers, seeded and chopped

2 Cups cooked black beans

1 small onion, chopped

2 Cups tomatoes, seeded and chopped

2 garlic cloves, minced

1/2 Cup rice vinegar

1/4 Cup olive oil

1/2 Teaspoon salt

1/4 Teaspoon pepper

Instructions

In a large bowl, place the couscous with boiling water.

Cover and wait until the couscous has absorbed all the water.

Add the remaining ingredients. Mix well and season with salt and pepper. Serve.

Brown Rice Greek Salad

Ingredients

1/2 Cup Brown rice, cooked

1/2 Cup white beans, canned, drained, rinsed

1/2 Cup fresh spinach

1/2 Cup tomatoes, no seeds

1/2 Cup English Cucumber, no seeds

1/4 Cup avocado, diced

1 Tablespoon red onion, chopped

2 Tablespoons Feta cheese, crumbled

2 Tablespoons extra virgin olive oil

1 Teaspoon red wine vinegar

To taste salt and pepper

Instructions

In a medium bowl, combine brown rice, beans, spinach, tomatoes, cucumber, avocado, onion, and cheese until combined.

Drizzle oil and vinegar on top and season to taste with salt and pepper and toss together.

Can be served alone or with whole wheat pita bread.

Cilantro Bean Salad

Ingredients

14 Ounces can kidney beans, drained and rinsed

14 Ounces can garbanzo beans, drained and rinsed

1 medium red onion, diced

1 small red bell pepper, seeded and chopped

1 Cup fresh cilantro

1/2 Cup balsamic vinegar

1 Tablespoon Dijon mustard

1 1/2 Teaspoon cumin

3 garlic cloves

1/2 Teaspoon salt

1 1/2 Cup olive oil

1/2 lemon, juiced

Instructions

In a medium bowl, combine beans, onion and bell pepper and set aside.

In a food processor, blend the rest of the ingredients until smooth. Pour half of the dressing over bean mixture and combine.

Refrigerate at least one hour. Pour remaining dressing over salad and mix gently just before serving. Serve at room temperature.

Fruit Salad with Avocado

Ingredients

2 large avocados, pitted and diced

1 peach, unpeeled, pitted and diced

1 apple, unpeeled, cored and diced

1 Cup cantaloupe, chopped

1 shallot, chopped finely

1 English cucumber, seedless, chopped

1/4 Cup fresh lime juice

1/4 Cup fresh mint, chopped

8 large lettuce leaves

Instructions

In a medium bowl, combine all ingredients except the lettuce leaves.

Sprinkle with lime juice and mint and toss together to combine.

Let the salad sit at least 10-20 minutes. Serve over 2 leaves of lettuce per serving.

Garbanzo and Tomato Salad

Ingredients

4 Ounces medium tomatoes, seeded and chopped

28 Ounces can garbanzo beans, drained and rinsed

1/4 Cup red onion, chopped finely

1 Cup Italian parsley, chopped finely

2 Tablespoons lemon juice

1/4 Cup olive oil

1/2 Teaspoon salt

1/4 Teaspoon pepper

Instructions

In a large bowl, combine tomatoes, garbanzo beans, onions and fresh parsley. Set aside.

In a separate small bowl whisk together lemon juice, olive oil and salt. Pour dressing over vegetables. Mix and serve.

Greek White Bean and Feta Salad

Ingredients

2 Tablespoons plain yogurt

3 Tablespoons olive oil

2 Tablespoons fresh lemon juice

3/4 Teaspoons oregano

1 Tablespoon fresh mint, chopped

28 Ounces white cannellini beans, drained and rinsed

1/2 Cup red onion, chopped finely

3 medium tomatoes, seeded and chopped

1/4 Cup Greek olives, pitted

1/2 Cup feta cheese, crumbled

2 Cups fresh spinach leaves, torn

Instructions

In large bowl, combine yogurt, olive oil, lemon juice, oregano, and mint; whisk well.

Add beans, onion, tomato, olives and feta cheese; toss lightly.

Refrigerate for at least one hour. Serve on a bed of spinach.

Green Bean Potato Salad

Ingredients

1 1/2 Pound fresh green beans

6 small red potatoes, unpeeled, cubed

1 small onion, thinly sliced

1/3 Cup olive oil

1/4 Cup red wine vinegar

1/4 Cup rice vinegar

1 Tablespoon garlic powder

1 Teaspoon sugar

Instructions

In a large pot of boiling water, cook green beans and potatoes about 7 minutes or until crisp-tender.

Drain and place only the beans in cold water to stop cooking process. Drain and set aside.

In a large salad bowl, combine green beans, potatoes and onions.

For dressing, in a small bowl, whisk together olive oil, vinegars, garlic powder and sugar.

Pour dressing over vegetables and toss to coat well. Refrigerate one hour prior to serving.

Green Bean Tuna Salad

Ingredients

3 Pounds green beans

1/2 Cup mayonnaise

1/3 Cup tarragon vinegar

1 Teaspoon Dijon mustard

Small shallots, sliced thinly

12 Ounces tuna fish, drained

Small sprigs tarragon, chopped finely

Instructions

In a large pot of boiling water, add green beans.

Reduce heat to low, cover and simmer 5-10 minutes until beans are tender.

Drain and place beans in cold water to stop cooking process. Drain and set aside.

In a large bowl, combine mayonnaise, vinegar and mustard. Add green beans, shallots and tuna fish; toss to coat with dressing.

Cover and refrigerate one hour prior to serving. Garnish with fresh tarragon and serve.

Grilled Shrimp and Bean Salad

Ingredients

1 1/2 Pound shrimp, peeled, cleaned, and deveined,

1/2 Cup olive oil

2 garlic cloves, minced

1/2 Teaspoon salt

2 small shallots, sliced thinly

1 Tablespoon fresh Italian parsley, chopped

1 1/2 Tablespoon fresh basil, chopped

1 Tablespoon red wine vinegar

28 Ounces white cannellini beans, drained and rinsed

Instructions

In a shallow glass dish, combine 1/4 cup of the olive oil with the garlic and 1/4 teaspoon of the salt. Add the shrimp and mix well. Set aside. In a medium bowl, combine the shallots with the remaining 1/4 cup oil and 1/4 teaspoon salt, parsley, basil, and vinegar. Gently stir in the beans.

Grill the shrimp over medium-high heat, turning once, until just done, about 3-5 minutes. Serve the shrimp with the bean salad.

Add the shrimp and mix well. Set aside.

In a medium bowl, combine the shallots with the remaining 1/4 cup oil and 1/4 teaspoon salt, parsley, basil, and vinegar.

Gently stir in the beans. Grill the shrimp over medium-high heat, turning once, until just done, about 3-5 minutes.

Serve the shrimp with the bean salad.

Light Shrimp and Barley Salad

Ingredients

1 Cup barley

2 Cups chicken broth

1/2 Cup shrimp, peeled, deveined, and cooked

1 medium green pepper, seeded and chopped

1 Teaspoon Dijon mustard

1/2 Cup mayonnaise

1/2 Cup fresh basil, chopped

Instructions

In a medium saucepan, bring barley and chicken broth to a boil. Reduce heat and simmer for 30 - 40 minutes, or until the barley is tender.

Drain well and fluff with a fork.

In a large serving bowl, combine the barley, shrimp, green pepper, mustard, mayonnaise and basil, and chill at least 30 minutes.

Garnish with fresh basil. Serve.

Mango Black Bean Salad

Ingredients

28 Ounces black beans, drained and rinsed

4 medium mangoes, peeled and diced

1 Cup fresh Italian parsley, chopped

2 small scallions, chopped finely

2 medium red peppers, seeded and diced

2 Tablespoons olive oil

1/2 Cup balsamic vinegar

1/4 Teaspoon salt

Instructions

In a large salad bowl, combine beans with mangoes, parsley, scallions, and red bell peppers.

In a separate small bowl, whisk together the oil, vinegar and salt. Pour over vegetables and mix well. Serve.

Mediterranean Salmon and Potato Salad

Ingredients

1 Pound red potatoes, unpeeled, cut into wedges

1/2 Cup olive oil

2 Tablespoons balsamic vinegar

1 Tablespoon rosemary, minced

2 Cups white cannellini beans, drained and rinsed

4 salmon fillets, 4 oz. each

2 Tablespoons lemon juice

1/4 Teaspoon salt

8 large lettuce leaves, torn

2 Cups English cucumber, seedless, sliced

Instructions

In a medium saucepan, bring water to a boil and cook potatoes until tender, about 10 minutes. Drain and pour potatoes back into pan.

To make dressing, in a small bowl, whisk together 1/2 cup of olive oil, vinegar and rosemary. Combine potatoes and white beans with dressing. Set aside.

In a separate medium pan, heat the remaining 2 tbsp. of olive oil over medium-high heat. Add salmon fillets and sprinkle with lemon juice and salt. Cook about 5-7 minutes on each side or until fish flakes easily.

To serve, place lettuce and cucumber slices on a serving platter top with potato salad and fish fillets.

Quick Spinach and Black Bean Salad

Ingredients

2 Cups black beans, cooked, drained, and rinsed

1/4 Cup green onions, chopped finely

10 Ounces fresh spinach

Red pepper, seeded, and chopped

Yellow pepper, seeded and chopped

1/2 Cup feta, crumbled

1 Cup Italian dressing

Instructions

In a medium bowl, combine beans, onions, spinach, peppers and cheese.

Pour dressing on top and mix together until combined

Shrimp, Pasta and Spinach Salad

Ingredients

1/2 Pound whole wheat pasta

3/4 Pounds medium shrimp, cooked

2 Cups fresh spinach

Roma tomatoes, seeded and chopped

1/2 Cup Ranch salad dressing

4 Tablespoons fresh basil, chopped

1/4 Cup Parmesan cheese, grated

Instructions

Bring a large pot of salted water to a boil. Cook pasta according to package instructions until al dente. Drain.

While pasta is cooking, in a large bowl, combine shrimp, spinach, tomatoes, salad dressing and cooked pasta.

Refrigerate for 20 minutes. Toss together with basil and cheese. Serve.

DIVERTICULITIS-FRIENDLY HIGH FIBER RECIPES

Apple Chicken Pita Pocket

Ingredients

Chicken cooked (boiled/grilled)

Unpeeled apples

Yoghurt

Lettuce leaves

Pita bread

Any other preferred vegetable

Salt and pepper to taste

Instructions

In a bowl add all the ingredients and mix well.

Fill the pita pocket and serve.

Baked Salmon with Vegetable Quinoa

Ingredients

1 salmon fillet

Salt, and pepper as per taste

Olive oil 2 tbsp.

Half cup quinoa

1 cup vegetable broth

1 small diced onion

Garlic as per taste

Bell pepper diced

Dices Zucchini

Fresh parsley

Lemon juice as per taste

Instructions

Set the oven's temperature to 375°F (190°C).

Add salt and pepper to the salmon fillet.

Over medium heat, warm the olive oil in a skillet. Salmon fillets should be added and cooked for two to three minutes on each side, or until golden.

Place the fish on a baking dish and cook it in the preheated oven for 8 to 10 minutes, depending on how done you want your salmon.

In the meanwhile, drain the quinoa after rinsing it in a fine mesh sieve.

Bring the vegetable broth to a boil in a saucepan. Regain the boil after adding the quinoa. For 18 to 20 minutes, or until the quinoa is cooked and the stock has been absorbed, reduce the heat to low, cover, and simmer.

Sauté the bell pepper, zucchini, onion, and garlic in the same pan until they are tender.

Add the parsley, cooked quinoa, and lemon juice by stirring.

Serve the veggie quinoa beside the baked fish.

Grilled Chicken Breast with Mashed Potatoes and Steamed Carrot

Ingredients

Boneless, skinless chicken breast is preferred

1 large potato, peeled and diced

1 tablespoon unsalted butter

1/4 cup low-fat milk

Salt and pepper to taste

1 cup steamed carrots

Instructions

Preheat the grill or grill pan over medium heat.

Season the chicken breast with salt and pepper.

Grill the chicken breast until fully cooked, with an internal temperature of 165°F (74°C). Cooking time may vary depending on the thickness of the chicken breast.

While the chicken is grilling, boil the diced potatoes in a pot of water until they are soft and easily mashed.

Drain the potatoes and transfer them back to the pot. Add butter, milk, salt, and pepper.

Mash the potatoes until smooth and creamy.

Steam the carrots until tender.

Serve the grilled chicken breast with a side of mashed potatoes and steamed carrots.

Apple and Pear Pita Pockets

Ingredients

1/2 small apple, unpeeled, chopped

1/2 small pear, unpeeled, chopped

1/4 Cup cottage cheese

1 whole wheat pita bread

Instructions

Combine the apple, pear, and cottage cheese in a bowl.

Slice the pita bread to make a pocket. Fill the pocket with the fruit mixture.

Sprinkle some cinnamon or drizzle a little honey or agave syrup for added sweetness.

Apple Raisin Pancakes

Ingredients

2 eggs

1 Cup unsweetened applesauce

1 Teaspoon cinnamon

2 Teaspoons brown sugar

1 Cup wheat flour

1/2 Cup white flour

2 Teaspoons baking powder

2 Teaspoons vanilla

1/2 Cup golden, seedless raisins

Non-stick cooking spray

1 Cup milk

Instructions

In a medium bowl, beat eggs until fluffy.

Add applesauce, cinnamon, sugar, flours, baking powder, vanilla and raisins and continue to stir just until smooth.

Heat griddle or pan over medium heat. Spray with non-stick cooking spray. For each pancake, pour about 1/4 cup of batter into hot pan.

Cook pancakes until edges get puffy. Turn and cook other side until golden. Serve pancakes with additional applesauce if desired.

Apricot Honey Oatmeal

Ingredients

1 Cup water or milk or almond milk

1/4 Cup dried apricots, chopped

1/2 Cup rolled oats

1 Tablespoon honey

1/4 Teaspoon cinnamon

Instructions

Place water or milk, apricots, honey, and cinnamon and oats in a microwave-safe bowl.

Cook in microwave for about 2 minutes until most of the liquid is absorbed, stirring occasionally.

Asparagus and Bean Frittata

Ingredients

2 Tablespoons olive oil

1 Cup onion, chopped

1 Cup red pepper, seeded, chopped

1 garlic clove, minced

14 Ounces can red or black or white beans, drained, rinsed

1 Cup asparagus, cooked and chopped

4 eggs

1/2 Teaspoon salt

1/4 Cup Parmesan cheese

Instructions

Preheat oven to 350 degrees.

In a large oven-proof pan, heat 1 tbsps. olive oil over medium-high heat. Cook onions, red peppers, garlic, and red beans until vegetables are soft (about 10 minutes). Set aside.

In medium bowl, beat eggs and salt, then add asparagus; set aside.

Add remaining 1 tbsps. olive oil into the vegetable pan and pour in the egg mixture. Reduce heat to medium-low and cook for 10 to 15 minutes, or until mixture is set on bottom and lightly browned.

Sprinkle Parmesan cheese over top of mixture and broil in the oven for an additional 3 to 5 minutes or until cheese is lightly browned and eggs are cooked through.

Banana Bran Muffins

Ingredients

1 1/2 Cup All-Bran cereal

2/3 Cups milk

4 eggs

1/4 Cup canola oil

1 Cup ripe banana, mashed (about 2 bananas)

1/2 Cup brown sugar

1 Cup whole wheat flour

2 Teaspoons baking powder

1/2 Teaspoon salt

Instructions

Preheat oven to 400F degrees.

In a large bowl, combine All-Bran cereal and milk and set aside. Add eggs and oil; stir in mashed banana and brown sugar and combine well.

In a separate small bowl, combine flour, baking powder and salt. Add dry ingredients to banana mixture, stirring just until combined.

Pour batter evenly into 12 greased or paper-lined muffin tins; Bake 15 to 18 minutes or until golden-brown and firm. Allow to cool prior to serving.

Banana Breakfast Smoothie

Ingredients

1 medium banana

1 Cup milk, almond or regular

1/2 Cup plain yogurt

1/4 Cup 100% Bran flakes

1 Teaspoon vanilla extract

2 Teaspoons honey or agave syrup

1/2 Cup ice

1 Pinch cinnamon

1 Pinch nutmeg

Instructions

Combine all ingredients in a blender and process on medium speed until smooth.

Garnish with cinnamon and/or nutmeg.

Bran Muffins

Ingredients

2 Cups All-Bran cereal

1/4 Cup brown sugar

1/2 Cup butter

2 eggs

2 Cups buttermilk

2 1/2 Cups whole wheat flour

2 1/2 Teaspoons baking soda

1/2 Teaspoon salt

1 Cup dates

1 Cup seedless raisins

Instructions

Preheat oven to 400F degrees.

Soak 1 cup of All-Bran cereal in 1 cup boiling water and set aside. In a mixer, cream sugar and butter together until well blended. Add eggs, one at a time and beat until fluffy. Add buttermilk and soaked bran mixture.

In a separate bowl, combine flour, baking soda, and salt. Add flour mixture into the batter but do not over mix. Add in remaining 1 cup of cereal, dates and raisins. Pour batter evenly into 10 greased or paper-lined muffin tins.

Bake 15-20 minutes. Allow to cool prior to serving.

Soak 1 cup of All-Bran cereal in 1 cup boiling water and set aside.

In a mixer, cream sugar and butter together until well blended. Add eggs, one at a time and beat until fluffy. Add buttermilk and soaked bran mixture.

In a separate bowl, combine flour, baking soda, and salt. Add flour mixture into the batter but do not over mix. Add in remaining 1 cup of cereal, dates and raisins.

Pour batter evenly into 10 greased or paper-lined muffin tins. Bake 15-20 minutes. Allow to cool prior to serving.

Breakfast Carrot Cake

Ingredients

1 1/3 Cup water

1/2 Cup brown sugar

1 Cup seedless raisins

2 carrots, grated

1 apple, unpeeled, chopped

1 Teaspoon cinnamon

1 Teaspoon ground cloves

1 Teaspoon nutmeg

2 Teaspoons butter

2 Cups whole wheat flour

1 Teaspoon baking soda

Instructions

Preheat oven to 375F degrees. Spray a 9x5 inch loaf pan with non-stick cooking spray.

In a medium saucepan, over low heat, mix together water, sugar, raisins, carrots, apples, cinnamon, cloves, nutmeg, and butter. Cook for 5-7 minutes, until well combined, and sugar dissolves. Remove pan from heat and allow to cool.

In a large bowl, combine flour, baking soda and salt. Stir carrot mixture into flour mixture and mix just until combined.

Pour into prepared pan. Bake for 1 1/4 hours, or until a knife inserted in the center comes out clean. Cool on wire rack.

Broccoli Omelet

Ingredients

8 eggs

4 Tablespoons milk

1/2 Teaspoon salt

1 1/2 Tablespoon extra-virgin olive oil

1/2 onion, chopped

1 Cup broccoli, fresh or frozen and thawed

1/2 Cup Monterrey Jack cheese, shredded

Instructions

In a bowl, whisk together eggs, milk and salt.

Heat olive oil in a medium skillet over medium-high heat, add onion and broccoli and cook until tender, about 7 minutes. Add the egg mixture, stirring to cook eggs evenly.

Sprinkle with cheese. Lower heat and cover until cheese melts. Flip over in half and serve.

Carrot and Zucchini Bread

Ingredients

3 1/2 Cups whole wheat flour

1 Tablespoon baking powder

1 Teaspoon baking soda

1/2 Teaspoon salt

1 Teaspoon cinnamon

2 eggs, lightly beaten

1 1/2 Cup buttermilk

2 Tablespoons butter, melted

1/2 Cup brown sugar

1 Cup zucchini, unpeeled, grated

1 Cup carrot, grated

1 Cup apple, unseeded, grated

Instructions

Preheat oven to 350F degrees.

Spray two 9x5-inch loaf pans with non-stick cooking spray. In a bowl, combine the flour, baking powder, baking soda, salt, and cinnamon; set aside.

In a large, separate bowl, combine the eggs, buttermilk, and melted butter. Stir in the brown sugar. Add the zucchini, carrots, and apple and combine.

Stir in the dry ingredients into the wet ingredients and stir gently until just combined.

Pour batter into prepared loaf pans. Bake for 60 minutes, or until a knife inserted into the center of the loaf comes out clean. Cool loaves in the pan for 10 minutes before removing to a wire rack to cool completely.

Pumpkin Pie Oatmeal

Ingredients

1/2 Cup rolled oats

3/4 Cups milk or water

1/2 Cup pumpkin puree

1 Teaspoon brown sugar

1 Teaspoon pumpkin spice

Instructions

In a microwave-safe bowl, mix together oats, milk or water and pumpkin puree.

Cook in microwave on high for 45 seconds. Stir and microwave for another 30 seconds.

Sprinkle with brown sugar and pumpkin spice and add a splash of milk.

Santé Fe Omelet

Ingredients

4 eggs

2 Tablespoons milk or water

1/4 Teaspoon salt

1 1/2 Tablespoon butter

1/2 Cup red beans, drained, rinsed

1 tomato, seeded, chopped

1/2 Cup green bell pepper, seeded, chopped

2 Tablespoons cheddar cheese, grated

2 Pieces whole wheat tortillas

Instructions

In a medium bowl, whisk together eggs, milk or water and salt.

Heat butter in a medium skillet and add red beans. Cook for 3 minutes, add tomatoes and green peppers.

Cook for another 5 minutes until vegetables soften. Pour in egg mixture and sprinkle the cheese over the eggs.

Cover until cheese melts. Serve with whole wheat tortillas.

Sunrise Burrito Wrap

Ingredients

1 Tablespoon olive oil

2 Slices turkey

1/4 Cup green bell pepper, seeded, chopped

1/4 Cup black beans

2 eggs

2 Tablespoons milk

1/4 Teaspoon salt

2 Tablespoons Monterrey Jack cheese, grated

1 whole wheat tortilla

Instructions

In a small non-stick pan, heat olive oil on medium heat and cook turkey about 2 minutes until slightly crispy.

Add bell peppers and beans and continue to cook until warmed through.

In a small bowl beat together egg with milk and salt.

Add beaten eggs and stir gently until eggs are almost cooked through.

Add grated cheese and lower heat to lowest setting.

Cover and continue to cook until cheese has completely melted. Place mixture on wheat tortilla and roll into a burrito.

Tropical Fruit Smoothie

Ingredients

1 Cup mix of mangoes, pineapples, bananas

1 Cup plain or vanilla yogurt

1/2 Cup All Bran cereal

1 Teaspoon vanilla

1 Tablespoon honey, or agave nectar, optional

1 Cup almond or coconut milk or water

1/2 avocado

1 Cup ice

Instructions

Combine all ingredients in a blender and process on high speed until smooth and creamy.

Zucchini and Bean Scramble

Ingredients

2 Tablespoons olive oil

1/2 Cup red onions, chopped finely

1 medium zucchini, seeded, chopped

14 Ounces can black beans, drained, rinsed

1/2 tomato, seeded, chopped

4 eggs

1/4 Cup milk

1 Teaspoon salt

4 whole wheat English muffins

Instructions

In a large non-stick pan, heat olive oil over moderate heat.

Add onions, zucchini, black beans and tomato. Cook for 5-10 minutes or until vegetables are soft.

In a separate bowl, mix together eggs and milk and salt. Add egg mixture to pan and stir to cook through, about 5 minutes.

Serve with whole wheat English muffins.

DIVERTICULITIS-FRIENDLY HEALTHY SNACKS

Baked Sweet Potato Fries

Ingredients

4 small sweet potatoes, unpeeled

1 Tablespoon butter, melted

1/4 Teaspoon salt

Dash of nutmeg

Instructions

Preheat oven to 450F degrees.

Spray a large baking pan with non-stick cooking spray.

Scrub potatoes and cut lengthwise into quarters, then cut each quarter into 2 wedges.

Arrange potatoes in a single layer in pan.

In a small bowl, combine butter, salt, and nutmeg.

Brush mixture onto potatoes and coat evenly.

Bake in oven 20 minutes or until brown and tender.

Citrus Carrots

Ingredients

1 Pound baby carrots

2 Tablespoons balsamic vinegar

1/2 Cup orange juice

1 orange, peeled and chopped

1 Tablespoon green onions, chopped finely

1 Tablespoon fresh dill, chopped

Instructions

Steam carrots in a steamer until tender or plunge carrots into boiling water and cook for about 10 - 12 minutes until tender. Drain. Rinse with cold water and drain again.

In a medium bowl, combine carrots, vinegar and orange juice. Stir to combine. Add orange segments, onions and dill. Lightly toss and serve.

Greek Lettuce Wraps

Ingredients

1/4 Cup mayonnaise

2 Teaspoons lemon juice

1/2 Cup white beans, drained and rinsed

1/3 Cup feta cheese, crumbled

2 Tablespoons pimentos, chopped

8 large lettuce leaves

1/2 Pound cooked chicken breast, cubed

Instructions

In a medium bowl, combine mayonnaise and lemon juice.

Stir in beans, mashing slightly with fork. Add cheese and pimentos, and mix lightly.

Spread lettuce leaves evenly with bean mixture. Top with chicken; roll up. Serve.

Honey Baked Apples

Ingredients

4 apples, unpeeled

1/4 Cup brown sugar

1/2 Teaspoon ground cloves

1/2 Teaspoon cinnamon

1/2 Cup honey

1/2 Cup water

Instructions

Preheat oven to 400 degrees.

Core and slice apples into 1/2" rings. Place them in a shallow baking dish for later use.

In a small saucepan, combine and heat brown sugar, cloves, cinnamon, honey and water.

Pour over apples and bake 15 minutes or until tender, turning to baste once or twice. Serve.

Kidney Bean Salsa

Ingredients

14 Ounces red kidney beans, drained and rinsed

2 tomatoes, seeded and chopped

1 yellow bell pepper, seeded and chopped

1 avocado, chopped

1 Tablespoon cilantro, chopped

2 Tablespoons lime juice

1/4 Teaspoon salt

Instructions

In large bowl, mix all ingredients until combined well.

Serve with warm tortillas or whole wheat chips.

Oatmeal Chocolate Chip Cookies

Ingredients

1/3 Cup brown sugar

1/2 Cup butter, softened

1/2 Teaspoon vanilla extract

1 egg

1 Cup whole grain, rolled oats

3/4 Cups whole wheat flour

1/2 Teaspoon baking soda

1/2 Cup dark chocolate chips

Instructions

Heat oven to 350 degrees. In a large bowl, cream brown sugar and butter until well combined. Stir in vanilla and egg and mix until light and fluffy. Stir in rolled oats, whole wheat flour, baking soda and fold in chocolate chips. Onto a cookie sheet covered with a Silpat mat or foil, drop the dough by rounded tablespoons (you can also use an ice cream scooper) about 2 inches apart.

Bake 10-12 minutes or until golden brown. Cool slightly; remove from cookie sheet to a wire rack.

White Bean Puree

Ingredients

14 Ounces cannellini beans, drained and rinsed

2 garlic cloves

1/4 Cup fresh Italian parsley

1/2 lemon, juiced

1/4 Teaspoon oregano

1/2 Teaspoon salt

1/3 Cup olive oil

Instructions

Blend all ingredients in a food processor until almost smooth. Serve with crusty bread, whole wheat crackers, or fresh vegetables

Baked Artichoke Dip

Ingredients

14 Ounces artichokes, drained and chopped

14 Ounces cannellini beans, drained and rinsed

1/2 Cup mayonnaise

1/2 Cup plain Greek yogurt

1 Cup Parmesan cheese, grated

10 Ounces frozen spinach, thawed and chopped

1/2 Cup red bell pepper, seeded and chopped

1/4 Cup Mozzarella cheese, shredded

Instructions

Heat oven to 350ºF. Mix artichokes, beans, mayonnaise, Greek yogurt, and Parmesan cheese. Stir in spinach and bell pepper.

Spoon mixture into 1-quart casserole. Sprinkle with Mozzarella cheese.

Cover and bake about 20 minutes or until cheese is melted. Serve warm with vegetables or whole wheat baguette slices.

Spinach and Mushroom Toss

Ingredients

2 Teaspoons olive oil

1/4 Cup shallots, minced

3 garlic cloves, minced

3 bacon strips, chopped

4 Cups white mushrooms, sliced

3 Tablespoons balsamic vinegar

1 1/2 Tablespoon low sodium soy sauce

20 Ounces fresh baby spinach

Instructions

In a large pan, heat olive oil over medium heat.

Add shallots and garlic and cook for 1 minute.

Add bacon and cook an additional 2-3 minutes, or until browned.

Add mushrooms and cook 3 to 5 minutes, until mushrooms are tender.

Add balsamic vinegar and soy sauce and bring to a simmer.

Add spinach and simmer 1 to 2 minutes, until spinach wilts, turning frequently.

CHAPTER VI: BEYOND THE PLATE: LIFESTYLE STRATEGIES FOR DIVERTICULITIS MANAGEMENT

To help prevent recurring flare-ups, a common occurrence in about one-third of patients with uncomplicated diverticulitis, we suggest:

Increase Fiber Intake:

A beneficial dietary approach for diverticulitis is focusing on a high-fiber diet. Increase plenty of fiber-rich foods like:

- Leafy greens
- Cooked and raw vegetables
- Low-glycemic fruits

- Whole grains
- Nuts and seeds

Eliminate Unhealthy Foods:

Avoid junk food, processed items, and white flours and grains. Transition gradually to a Mediterranean diet or another healthy eating plan that emphasizes vitamin- and mineral-rich vegetables and fiber. Rapidly increasing fiber intake may lead to gas, potentially irritating your gut lining and triggering a flare.

The dietary adjustments serve two primary purposes: **firstly, providing your body with essential nutrients to support optimal organ function, including your gut, without discomfort. Secondly, promoting regular and comfortable bowel movements.**

Facilitate Bowel Movements:

Respond promptly to the urge to defecate rather than suppressing it. Constipation and retained fecal matter can exacerbate diverticulitis symptoms. Maintain adequate hydration to ensure soft and easily passable stools.

If your diet lacks fiber or fluids, constipation may cause painful bowel movements and aggravate gut irritation. Consider adding prunes or prune juice if your fiber intake is insufficient or if you struggle with constipation despite a high-fiber diet.

You may also try adding one teaspoon of ground psyllium seeds to a glass of liquid, consuming the mixture before it thickens. Additionally, over-the-counter stool softeners containing polyethylene glycol can be beneficial. Avoid products containing senna, as they can be habit-forming and irritate the gut lining. However, it's essential not to rely on stool softeners long-term.

Add in more exercise

In addition to fiber, water, and stool softeners, regular exercise can facilitate bowel movements. Exercise not only strengthens your arm, leg, and core muscles but also tones the muscles in your intestines, promoting more comfortable and regular stool passage.

If you've been inactive, begin with a daily walk and gradually increase the duration to 30 minutes. Progress by incorporating more intensity and variety into your exercise routine. Include resistance training and flexibility-enhancing techniques. Always consult your doctor before making changes to your exercise regimen.

Seek Appropriate Assistance:

While lifestyle modifications can mitigate the risk of diverticulitis complications, if you're experiencing pain, relief shouldn't be delayed. If lifestyle adjustments and medications prove ineffective, surgery to remove damaged intestinal sections may be necessary.

During a flare-up, focus on consuming clear broths and other non-irritating liquids to nourish yourself without aggravating your gut. Symptoms of a flare include nausea, vomiting, abdominal pain, fever, chills, diarrhea, or constipation. You may require antibiotics to treat the infection and other medications for comfort while your gut heals.

Move It or Lose It: Exercise Essentials

Research indicates that *exercise holds significant benefits for individuals managing diverticulitis by enhancing digestive function, alleviating stress, and bolstering overall physical and mental well-being.* Additionally, exercise can aid in weight management, potentially lowering the risk of diverticulitis onset.

A study highlighted in the Journal of Gastrointestinal and Liver Diseases showcased that regular physical activity could diminish the likelihood of developing diverticulitis by up to 27%. Moreover, exercise has demonstrated efficacy in alleviating common symptoms such as abdominal discomfort, bloating, and constipation associated with diverticulitis.

However, it's imperative for individuals with diverticulitis to consult their healthcare provider before embarking on an exercise regimen, particularly those with severe or active cases who may need to postpone physical activity until inflammation diminishes.

For those with diverticulitis, *low-impact exercises like walking, swimming, or yoga are advisable as they enhance circulation and reduce stress without exerting undue pressure on the affected area.* Integrating physical activity into daily routines not only enhances overall fitness but also fortifies the immune system, particularly beneficial for individuals managing chronic conditions like diverticulitis.

Incorporating physical activity isn't solely advantageous for diverticulitis management; it offers a plethora of health benefits for everyone. Regular exercise promotes cardiovascular health, mitigates the risk of chronic ailments, and enhances mental well-being. Therefore, discuss with your healthcare provider about integrating exercise into your diverticulitis management plan to reap its multifaceted advantages.

Furthermore, engaging in *vigorous activities such as jogging, swimming laps, or playing tennis, alongside exercises that elevate heart rate and respiration (like brisk walking), is associated with decreased risks of diverticulitis and diverticular bleeding.* Additionally, such exercises are believed to foster a diverse population of beneficial gut microbes, contributing to healthy aging and longevity.

Stress Less, Live More: Stress Management Techniques

Stress is widely recognized as a catalyst for various illnesses due to its significant impact on the body, potentially contributing to the development of diverticulitis. Environmental factors play a pivotal role in around 60% of these cases. *The digestive system can be particularly vulnerable to stress, especially with a diet low in fiber or high in fat, both of which are known triggers for this inflammatory condition,* more prevalent among older individuals than younger ones.

While the precise connection between stress and diverticulitis isn't fully elucidated, stress-induced inflammation is considered a contributing factor. Elevated stress levels can disrupt bodily functions and digestive processes, mimicking the body's response to a physical threat, diverting essential resources away from vital areas and potentially leading to health issues.

Addressing this stress-induced medical condition involves various strategies:

Relaxation: Incorporate daily relaxation practices into your routine. Engage in meditation using a calming mantra like "Peace. Love. Hope" to alleviate anxiety and potentially rewire your brain to reduce stress responses.

Breathing Techniques: Practice slow, deep breathing exercises to reduce stress levels, lower heart rate, and alleviate hypertension.

Mindfulness: Embrace the present moment amidst busy schedules. Take pauses to appreciate your surroundings, weather, and personal feelings. Focusing on the present fosters gratitude and diminishes stress by grounding you in the here and now.

Connect with Friends: Schedule some time to meet with friends or have a phone call to alleviate stress. Building a sense of community and socializing can effectively reduce anxiety. Having a supportive circle of friends is essential for maintaining a healthy lifestyle.

Relax and De-Stress: Apply a heating pad to your back and shoulders for about 10 minutes to relieve tension and pain in these areas. Focus on relaxing each part of your body during this time. Aromatherapy with scented candles can also contribute to easing anxiety.

Find Humor: Laughter can be a powerful stress-reliever, lowering cortisol levels and boosting mood by releasing endorphins. Incorporate some laughter into your day to alleviate stress and improve overall well-being.

Listen to Music: Music has proven stress-reducing effects, helping to lower blood pressure and feelings of nervousness. Relaxing sounds like ocean waves or rainfall can be particularly soothing.

Get Moving: Engage in at least 30 minutes of exercise daily, whether it's trying a new activity like yoga or simply going for a run with your dog. Exercise is a natural anxiety and depression fighter.

Practice Gratitude: Keep a gratitude journal to remind yourself of your blessings, especially during challenging times. Reflecting on these blessings can uplift your mood and reduce stress.

Eat Healthy: Adhering to a diverticulitis-friendly diet can support overall health and stress reduction. Avoid turning to junk food during stressful moments and instead focus on nourishing options like broths, fruit juices, and low-fiber foods. Gradually reintroduce high-fiber foods after the initial healing phase.

Prioritize Sleep: Sufficient sleep is crucial for managing stress levels. Create a bedtime routine that promotes relaxation, such as lighting candles and avoiding electronics before bed. Aim for 7-9 hours of uninterrupted sleep each night, and consider napping during the day if needed to make up for lost sleep.

CHAPTER VII: BEFORE YOU GO, HERE'S A FINAL REMINDER!

If diverticula in your colon remain uninfected and free from inflammation, it's diagnosed as diverticulosis. However, when these pouches lead to symptoms such as abdominal pain and bloating, the condition is termed *Symptomatic Uncomplicated Diverticular Disease* (SUDD).

Bladder diverticula represent another form of this condition, occurring when pouches form in the bladder lining, protruding through weak areas in the bladder wall. While some bladder diverticula are congenital, others develop later in life due to blockages or bladder dysfunction caused by various factors, including illness or injury.

In cases where bladder diverticula become inflamed, diagnosed as bladder diverticulitis, treatment typically involves antibiotics and pain management. Surgery might be recommended for diverticula repair.

Furthermore, severe cases of diverticulitis in the colon can lead to complications involving the bladder, such as the formation of a colovesical fistula, connecting the colon and bladder. This condition requires medical attention to address its implications.

Diverticula can also manifest in the esophagus, albeit rarely. This occurs when pouches emerge in the esophageal lining, often developing gradually over an extended period. As they enlarge, they may trigger symptoms like difficulty swallowing, pain during swallowing, halitosis, regurgitation of food and saliva, pulmonary aspiration, and aspiration pneumonia.

Inflammation of esophageal diverticula is referred to as esophageal diverticulitis. This condition requires proper management and medical intervention to alleviate symptoms and prevent complications.

To address esophageal diverticulitis, your physician may recommend a course of antibiotics and pain relief medications. In some cases, surgical intervention may be necessary to repair the diverticula. Seeking further details about your treatment options is advisable.

Age stands out as a primary risk factor for diverticulitis, with older individuals at a higher likelihood of developing this condition compared to younger counterparts. It's commonly observed in men under 50 and women aged 50 to 70.

Those who develop diverticula at a younger age may have an increased susceptibility to diverticulitis. Younger individuals also tend to have higher hospital admission rates for diverticulitis compared to older demographics.

Various potential risk factors for diverticulitis have been identified through research. Family history plays a significant role, with genetic factors contributing to approximately 40 to 50 percent of the overall risk.

Low levels of vitamin D have also emerged as a potential risk factor, as some studies suggest a correlation between higher vitamin D levels and reduced risk of diverticulitis. However, further investigation is necessary to fully understand this relationship.

Obesity has been linked to an increased risk of diverticulitis, with studies indicating that individuals with higher BMI and larger waist sizes are more susceptible. The mechanisms behind this association, possibly involving alterations in gut bacteria balance, warrant further research.

Physical inactivity is another factor potentially influencing the risk of diverticulitis, with studies suggesting that active individuals are less prone to developing the condition. However, additional research is needed to elucidate this connection further.

Moreover, the regular use of nonsteroidal anti-inflammatory drugs (NSAIDs) or smoking has been linked to an elevated risk of diverticulitis. Consistent use of aspirin, ibuprofen, or other NSAIDs may increase susceptibility, while smoking has been associated with a higher incidence of diverticular disease, including diverticulitis.

Based on a 2017 research review, there isn't substantial evidence indicating that alcohol consumption significantly increases the risk of diverticulitis. However, medical advice typically advocates for moderate alcohol intake. While excessive alcohol consumption may not directly trigger diverticulitis, it can contribute to various other health complications.

Certain risk factors associated with diverticulitis can potentially be mitigated through lifestyle adjustments. These include:

- Maintaining a moderate body weight
- Adopting a high-fiber diet to aid in stool bulk (although during acute diverticulitis episodes, high-fiber intake might be avoided)
- Limiting saturated fat intake
- Ensuring adequate vitamin D levels
- Engaging in regular physical activity whenever feasible
- Avoiding exposure to cigarette smoke

These preventive measures not only serves to reduce the risk of diverticulitis but also contributes to overall well-being.

Finding Support and Community along the Way: Seeking Guidance

If you're grappling with feelings of isolation or confusion amid changes in your health or caregiving responsibilities, community support groups can offer invaluable assistance. These groups provide a platform for individuals sharing similar health conditions, diagnoses, or caregiving experiences to connect and find solidarity. Typically informal in nature, they facilitate the exchange of personal stories, practical advice, and coping strategies relevant to the group's focus.

When seeking out a support group, there are various formats to explore. **In-person gatherings** may occur at local venues such as coffee shops, community centers, churches, schools, or libraries. They may have attendance limitations and could be either free or fee-based.

Virtual support groups, conducted online, offer broader accessibility, accommodating larger numbers of participants without geographical constraints. Usually, they are free to join and enable the hosting of multiple groups simultaneously due to the absence of physical space limitations.

Telephonic support groups operate through structured call-in sessions where participants share experiences or adopt a more flexible helpline-style approach. For instance, organizations like the

Alzheimer's Association offer round-the-clock helplines staffed by trained individuals to assist caregivers. Telephonic options suit those who may not feel ready for in-person group participation but still seek supportive resources.

To locate a suitable support group in your area, consider the type of group you prefer. *Disease- or diagnosis-specific groups can often be found through online associations related to the particular health condition.* Additionally, many healthcare facilities offer specialized support groups tailored to specific illnesses or caregiving challenges.

www.ingramcontent.com/pod-product-compliance
Lightning Source LLC
Chambersburg PA
CBHW050205230526
45470CB00001B/240